Cell Biology Research Progress

nova
Medicine & Health
New York

Cell Biology Research Progress

Dendritic Cell Biology as an Immune Dysfunction in Neoplasia
Lawrence M. Agius
2022. ISBN: 978-1-68507-486-9 (Softcover)
2022. ISBN: 978-1-68507-537-8 (eBook)

TRiPs Across Epithelial and Endothelial Barriers in Health and Disease
Alexander V. Zholos, PhD, DSc (Editor)
Ganna M. Tolstanova, PhD (Editor)
2021. ISBN: 978-1-68507-020-5 (Hardcover)
2021. ISBN: 978-1-68507-139-4 (eBook)

Na+K+-ATPase: Discovery, Functions and Regulation
Mohammed Awad Ali Khalid (Editor)
2021. ISBN: 978-1-53618-968-1 (Softcover)
2020. ISBN: 978-1-53619-050-2 (eBook)

A Closer Look at Membrane Proteins
Tristan B. Møller (Editor)
2020. ISBN: 978-1-53618-149-4 (Softcover)
2020. ISBN: 978-1-53618-538-6 (eBook)

Cadherins: Types, Structure and Functions
Jonathan McWilliam (Editor)
2020. ISBN: 978-1-53618-077-0 (Softcover)
2020. ISBN: 978-1-53618-096-1 (eBook)

More information about this series can be found at https://novapublishers.com/product-category/series/cell-biology-research-progress/

Amankeldi A. Salybekov, MD, PhD
Shuzo Kobayashi, MD, PhD
and Takayuki Asahara, MD, PhD
Editors

Endothelial Progenitor Cells in Health and Disease

nova
Medicine & Health
New York

DOI: https://doi.org/10.52305/ZZUL5783.

NOTICE TO THE READER

Library of Congress Cataloging-in-Publication Data

ISBN: 978-1-68507-794-5

Published by Nova Science Publishers, Inc. † New York

Contents

Preface

We are delighted to offer this textbook to the scientific community, entitled Endothelial Progenitor Cells in Health and Disease, which covers a timely topic in the rapidly evolving discipline of vascular biology. Written primarily for a life science audience and clinicians, the fundamentals of EPCs biology, and the latest characterization and definition in health and diseases are introduced, followed by explanations of the most cutting-edge cell therapy methods to cure ischemic diseases.

In section one, endothelial cell progenitor isolation methods and biological characterization were reported. The discovery of this novel endothelial progenitor cells (EPC) concept has overturned the previous dogma which suggested that vasculogenesis could only occur during embryogenesis. In fact, both vasculogenesis and angiogenesis may potentially have a synergistic role in postnatal revascularization. Also, this chapter summarized recent advances in EPC biology such as biological function, origin, definition, and classification. Each EPC culture and isolation method is clearly defined to prevent confusion in EPC biology. Section two focuses on EPC biological function alteration in cardiovascular diseases (CVD). Several large clinical trials have reported that the number and biological function are strongly associated with major adverse cardiovascular events. The diagnostic and prognostic potential of EPC is crucial in terms of CVD. In section three, biological dysfunction mechanisms of EPC and their scarcity in diabetic patients' peripheral blood was clearly described. Preclinical studies have shown that EPC-based therapy is feasible, safe, and efficacious in multiple disease states. Subsequently, this has led to several clinical trials demonstrating the feasibility and safety profile of EPC therapy against cardiovascular ischemic diseases. In section four, regenerative medicine pioneers discussed EPCs translation to the clinic and cell transplantation challenges along with their solutions. Personalized stem cell-based therapy approaches employing several clinical biomarkers, disease-related genetic-trait evaluation methods, and advanced analyses with state-of-the-art computational methods such as machine learning-based prediction can increase cell therapies' efficacy and decrease treatment costs. The last chapter in the book describes a therapeutic application of EPC-derived extracellular vesicles to cure CVD.

We would like to offer our acknowledgments to the all authors who contributed to the textbook chapters. Also, we would like to thank Ms. K. Kunita and the Nova Publishing group team for their immense assistance during this book edition.

Amankeldi A. Salybekov, MD, PhD
Shuzo Kobayashi, MD, PhD
Takayuki Asahara, MD, PhD
Febuary 2022,
Tokyo, Japan

Section I: EPC Biological Function and Origin

Chapter 1

Advances in Endothelial Progenitor Cell Biology

Amankeldi A. Salybekov, MD, PhD[1,2,3,*]
and Takayuki Asahara, MD, PhD[2]

[1]Kidney Disease and Transplant Center,
Shonan Kamakura General Hospital,
Kamakura, Japan
[2]Shonan Research Institute of Innovative Medicine,
Shonan Kamakura General Hospital,
Kamakura, Japan
[3] Qazaq Institute of Innovative Medicine,
Nur-Sultan, Kazakhstan

Abstract

Endothelial progenitor cells (EPCs) are currently being studied as the candidate cell sources for revascularization strategies. Despite these promising results, the widespread clinical acceptance of EPCs for clinical therapies remains hampered by several challenges. The challenges and issues surrounding the use of EPCs and the current strategies being developed to improve the harvest efficiency and functionality of EPCs for application in regenerative medicine are discussed. It has been observed that controversies emerged regarding the isolation techniques, classification, and origin of EPCs. This chapter attempts to highlight the concept of EPCs in a sequential manner from the speculative history to a definitive presence (origin, sources of EPCs, isolation, and identification techniques) and the significance of these EPCs. Additionally, this chapter is aimed at summarizing our current and future prospects regarding the

* Corresponding Author's Email: a.salybekov@shonankamakura.or.jp.

In: Endothelial Progenitor Cells in Health and Disease
Editors: Amankeldi A. Salybekov, Shuzo Kobayashi and Takayuki Asahara
ISBN: 978-1-68507-794-5

cross-talk of EPCs with the biology of hematopoietic cells and culture techniques in the context of regeneration-associated cells (RACs).

Keywords: endothelial progenitor cells, endothelial colony-forming cells, regeneration-associated cells, resident EPCs

Introduction

The discovery of endothelial progenitor cells (EPCs) shed light on the existence of postnatal vasculogenesis in humans [1, 2]. One year later, a laboratory showed evidence that a subset of $CD34^+$ cells have the capacity to differentiate into endothelial progenitor cells [3]. Since the discovery of EPCs, a large number of research studies have been accumulated regarding the biology of EPCs, origin, differentiation hierarchy, and also including translational animal studies and further clinical applications. However, this field has unresolved issues, such as ambiguous and controversial findings with regard to EPC biology and biological characteristics. This has facilitated the unification of EPC-related terminology based on the progress of recent research because of the important role of EPCs in vascular repair in health and disease and, in some cases, the progress toward use in cell therapy seemed to be a proper step forward in this area [4]. This chapter summarizes the current understanding of EPC biology, such as differentiation, origin, and the cross-talk between hematopoietic cells.

From Hemangioblasts to EPC

Hematopoietic stem cells (HSCs) in adults are believed to be derived from hemogenic endothelial cells (HECs) in mid-gestational embryos. Particularly, hematopoietic stem and progenitor cells (HSPCs) are visualized to emerge from aortic endothelial cells (ECs) (also known as the embryonic aorta-gonad-mesonephros (AGM) area) via a transient and dynamic process called the endothelial-to-hematopoietic transition to form intra-aortic hematopoietic clusters (IAHCs) [5-7]. Being located within the IAHCs or to the deeper sub-endothelial layers, pre-HSCs serve as the important cellular intermediates between HECs and HSCs, featured by their inducible repopulating capacity and priming with hematopoietic surface markers [5, 7]. Subsequently, based on the current concept of *de novo* generation of HSPC from the precursor of hemogenic endothelial cells, namely hemogenic angioblast or hemangioblasts, the latter is thought to migrate to, and propagate within, the fetal liver and fetal bone marrow as those tissues develop [5, 6, 8]. A previous mouse study identified that adult bone marrow-derived, phenotypically defined hematopoietic stem cells (c-kit+, Sca-1+, lineage–) give rise to functional endothelial cells [9]. Later, Case et al. isolated CD34+CD45-/+ cells and even further stringent selected for downstream EPCs markers like CD34+AC133+ VEGFR-2+ and assayed for either EPCs or HPCs colony forming-assay [10]. Notably, CD45+CD34+CD34+AC133+VEGFR-2+ cells formed HPCs colony but not EPCs, while CD45−CD34+ CD34+AC133+ VEGFR-2+ cells formed classical endothelial cells like morphology, and highly proliferative potential, and expressed the CD31 marker [10]. More recently, Ratajczak et al. described the successful isolation of very small embryonic-like stem cells (VSELs) from umbilical cord blood. Morphologically, VSELs are small cells, corresponding in size to the cells in the inner cell mass of the blastocyst, and, depending on the measurement conditions (in suspension or after adhesion to slides), they measure ≈ 3 to 5 μm in mice and ≈5 to 7 μm in humans. The authors defined that VSELs are at the top of the stem cell hierarchy in the normal bone marrow, negative expression of CD45 marker, giving rise to HSCs, mesenchymal stem cells, and EPCs [11].

Taken together, the accumulating results suggest that hemangioblasts can give rise to HSCs and EPCs. It seems that either peripheral blood or umbilical cord blood derived CD34+CD45- cells mainly composes hemangioblasts, and their number and proliferative or self-renewal capacity reduces in the elder population.

EPCs Characterization *Ex Vivo*

The term of "EPC" grouped several distinct cell subtypes since the first original findings, and some of them cannot be characterized as EPC due to their divergent biological function and contribution for neoangiogenesis, also lack of distinct delineating immunophenotype markers from other cell lineages, and origin. To this end, several groups of laboratories attempted to summarize all of EPC related terms to have a consensus statement on the endothelial progenitor nomenclature [12]. Notably, the consensus statement distinguishes proangiogenic cells from "true EPCs" for our better understanding; on the other hand, the statement does not cover whole terminologies which have been utilized in the scientific literature so far. Thus, we returned back to the original introduction of EPC and development stages along with endothelial outgrowth cells and tissue resident EPCs to group them appropriately and define markers to delignate EPCs from other cells.

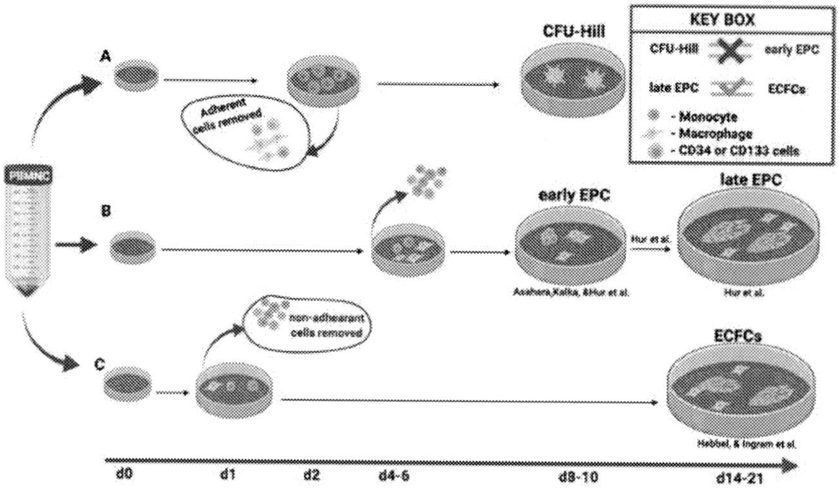

Figure 1. The methods of EPCs culture. Method A is colony formation units of Hill. In this method, the adherent cells were depleted at day 2/48 h due to the author's concern regarding the contamination by "circulating endothelial cells". Non-adherent cells were plated to the dish to count CFU-EC or CFU-Hill at day 5 to 9. Method B was developed to enhance EPC *ex vivo*. The non-adherent cells were discarded on days 4–6 while adherent cells further incubated up to day 10 in the studies of Kalka and Asahara et al. Subsequently, Hur et al. used the same method as Kalka et al. with slight modifications, such as the prolongation of incubation time. Notably, they observed endothelial outgrowth cells at day 14 in the midst of early EPC, which indicated that some of the hidden cells among an early EPC population can give rise to ECFCs. Thus, CD34+ and CD133+ cells depleted mononuclear cells could not form ECFC, whereas the presence of these cells successfully did. The last C method initially described by Hebbel et al. 1 day after plating the cells, non-adherent cells were removed. At days 14–21, the blood endothelial outgrowth cells appeared, morphologically and phenotypically similar to late EPC.

Initially, EPCs were characterized as CD34, KDR, and VE cadherin positive cells that were purified by magnetic beads. When these cells were plated on a fibronectin coated plate, they attached and expressed eNOS, Flk-1/KDR, and CD31, and finally released NO, indicating a full set of endothelial cell characteristics [13]. Taking into account that EPCs are extremely rare in circulating blood, to generate a sufficient number of cells, researchers have developed an *ex vivo* expansion culture system to expand rare EPCs using whole blood peripheral mononuclear cells (PBMCs). Kalka et al. introduced an *ex vivo* EPC expansion method using several growth factor cocktails [14]. The PBMCs were plated on culture dishes coated with human fibronectin for *4 days,* and then, nonadherent cells were discarded and *adherent or attached cells* were maintained by replacing the media in the culture for up to 10 days (Figure 1B). This culture technique facilitated the Hill et al. [15] group to develop a new growth media combination and to evaluate the endothelial cells colony forming unit (CFU-EC or also known as CFU-Hill) *in vitro* with significantly different protocols by utilizing PBMCs. The difference of CFU-Hill vs. Kalka is that PBMCs were resuspended in an endothelial growth medium and plated on fibronectin coated dishes for *48 hours* to avoid contamination by "*circulating endothelial cells*"; subsequently, *non-adherent* cells were seeded to another fibronectin coated dish for seven days to count the colonies (Figure 1A). Due to the ease-of-use, CFU-Hill produced a commercial kit to evaluate the EPC number, which was highly correlated with the Framingham cardiovascular risk factor score. However, several laboratories were concerned that these colonies were not "EPCs," and rather were mainly composed of myeloid and lymphoid cell subsets that were unable to form blood vessels in *in vivo* experiments [16] [17, 18]. Subsequently, Hur et al. [19] identified two types of EPC, namely *early* and *late,* by applying the same method as previously mentioned. The first media replacement occurred at *day 6*; thereafter, the media were changed every 3 days until late EPC appearance. Notably, after 2 weeks of plating, they observed distinct morphology colonies from early EPC, so-called late EPC, or ECFC in the midst of early EPC (Figure 1B and C). The early EPCs secrete more angiogenic cytokines or paracrine factors as the majority of them are composed of "circulating angiogenic cells" including monocyte/macrophages and lymphocytes, while late EPCs appeared two to three weeks after plating with a "cobblestone" morphology. In an animal study, both types of EPCs equally returned perfusion of the ischemic hindlimb (HLI) to levels that were similar to those recorded in the contralateral nonischemic hindlimb. Undoubtedly, the bona fide EPCs derived from the *rare heterogeneous CD34+ cells hidden in the early EPC populations* [19-21]. Over time, several controversial findings have accumulated in this field. Some authors claimed that CD34 or CD133 are not EPC markers [20], while other authors improperly or equally grouped early EPC and CFU-Hill culture techniques as the same method [12, 21] (Figure 1. see Key Box). Previous studies compared cord blood and PB derived CD34+ cells in the presence or absence of hematopoietic CD45 surface antigen expression between CFU-Hill vs. late EPCs, but not in the classical early EPC culture technique. This experiment concluded that CD34+CD45- cells generated late EPC while the CD34+CD45+ fraction did not; obviously, CFU-Hill may not form late EPC if attached cells were removed 48 hours after plating. Moreover, compelling evidence suggests that there is crosstalk between myeloid and lymphoid cells and EPC, which may exhibit EPC expansion [22]. Notably, our group and others have demonstrated that CD34 depleted either CB or PBMCs unable to generate any late EPC colonies or ECFCs, suggesting that late EPC are derived from CD34+ cells [23, 24].

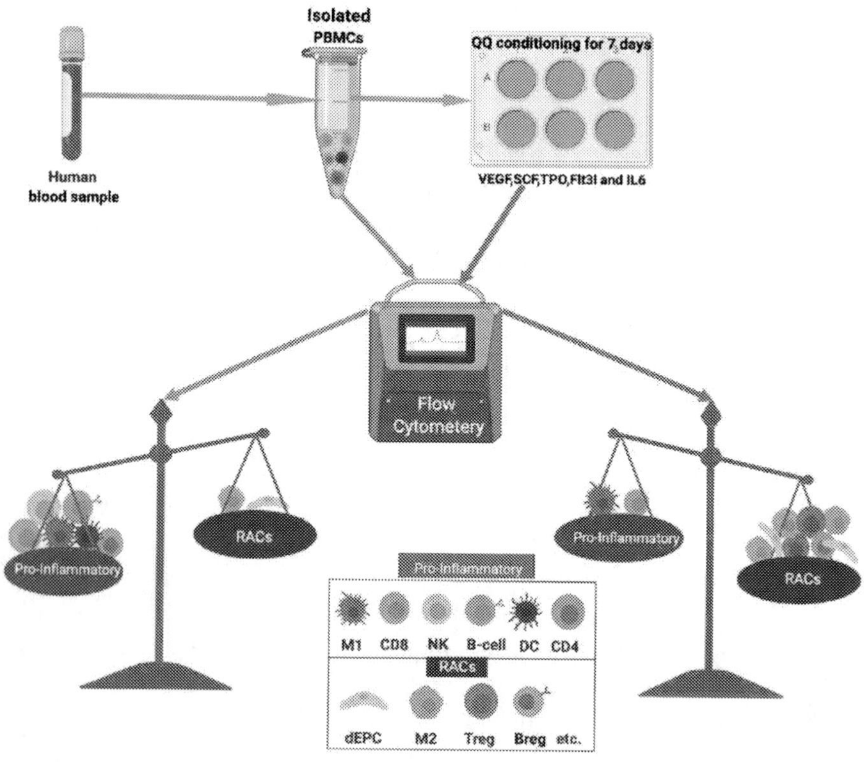

Figure 2. Regeneration-associated cells. PBMCs isolated and cultured in serum-free media with defined growth factor for 7 days. The pro-inflammatory cell phenotypes shift to anti-inflammatory cells in flow cytometry analysis.

Ex Vivo Culture Environment May Change the EPCs Surface Marker

Recently, Rossi et al. found the intracellular expression of CD133+ antigen marker in ECFCs [25]. When they transplanted CD133 molecule silenced ECFCs into HLI-induced mice, revascularization was significantly abolished, whilst the ECFCs transplantation was recovered, indicating that intracellular CD133 antigen expression is crucial for ECFC maintenance (25). Another report demonstrated that during cell culture, CD34- expressed ECFCs re-expressed CD34+. In addition, cell-cell contact formation and serum supplements significantly modulated the CD34 expressional profile. Functionally, these two populations are not identical; CD34+ ECFCs exhibited a higher tube-forming capacity and tip-cell gene expression rather than CD34- cells [26]. This result was consistent with the latest position paper on ECFCs, that recommends to the use of 10% FBS, instead of 5%. The latter significantly influences the ECFC colony formation ability [27]. The latest research studies on EPC also raised awareness on EPCs culturing on fibronectin or collagen types or on using fetal bovine serum; the latter releases extracellular vesicle cargo containing growth factors, mRNA, or miRNA, which may facilitate the proliferation and differentiation of cells, while their concentration is higher in the culture medium [28-32]. Another group also concerned regarding the functioning of such cells cultured endothelial CFU *in vivo* similar to the circulating cells. Thus, even single cell cultures with strict selection may not be excluded from the probability of *"reprogramming" in vitro* by an artificial milieu, which was reported formerly [21]. Taking into account the above issues, we have developed a clonogenic assay to address the primary circulating EPCs from different origin peripheral blood, bone marrow, and cord blood, respectively. From the single cord blood derived CD133+ cell, two types of colonies were raised at day 18 after plating into a semisolid culture dish, termed as small and large EPC-CFU. The large EPC-CFU was observed to highly express Ve- cadherin, vWF etc. and express CD45 and CD14 markers lesser in comparison with small EPC-CFU. Notably, the single-cell culture results indicated the presence of populations that can give rise to both endothelial and hematopoietic progenitors *in vitro* at a ratio of 24% without VEGF or 36% with VEGF, indicating that the growth factor may *"reprogram"* the cells. The hemato-endothelial commitment assay disclosed that large EPCs gained endothelial commitment and differentiation. Moreover, the transplantation of large EPCs markedly amplified the blood flow perfusion in the HLI model by the enhancement of the neovasculogenesis process [23].

Endothelial Colony-Forming Cells *(Ex Vivo)*

The origin and phenotype of blood endothelial outgrowth cells (BEOCs; which are also referred to as endothelial colony formation cells) was first described two decades ago by Lin et al. [33]. To address the origin of BEOC, isolation of samples of mononuclear cells from gender-mismatched bone marrow transplanted recipients and seeding to collagen type 1 coated plate was carried out. Consequently, unattached cells were removed after 24 h and only up to 19 endothelial like cells; 100–200 mononuclear cells were observed to remain on the plate. The latter showed a typical macrophage shape and died out three weeks later after plating. Morphologically, BEOCs were observed to have a "cobblestone" shape, highly positive for EPC/EC markers, such as CD34+, CD31+, VE-cadherin, CD146+, von Willebrand factor, CD31+, and negative expression for monocyte marker CD14+, respectively. Notably, upon a fluorescence *in situ* hybridization (FISH) analysis, the recipient genotype BEOC expansion was gradually decreased in the culture while donor-genotypes were dramatically increased by 1023-fold after 1 month, indicating that BOACs were derived from the bone marrow. Fujisawa et al. [34] investigated the origin of EPCs using the blood samples from sex-mismatched allogeneic bone marrow transplanted patients. The FISH analysis conformed that BOACs do not originate from the bone marrow, which is controversial to the findings of Lin et al. [33]. Subsequently, Ingram et al. [35] also identified endothelial outgrowth cells in culture between days 14 to 21, termed as "endothelial colony-forming cells (ECFCs)" derived from the human peripheral and umbilical cord blood. Therefore, this study utilized a clonogenic method to define the proliferative potential of EPCs at a single cell level as hinted by Lin et al. [36]. The *in vitro* study showed that ECFCs have a high proliferative potential as well as being clonally distinct from CFU-Hill, surface antigen expression of ECFCs close to EC while CFU-Hill contaminated with hematopoietic cell subsets (16). Consequently, several preclinical studies used ECFCs as a therapeutic cell source to cure several life-threatening diseases. The main dilemma in the widespread use of ECFCs are their scarcity in the peripheral blood, equating to 2.5 ECF colonies per milliliter of blood in healthy human subjects or even using advanced current culture techniques less than 70% of individuals may form ECFCs colonies

[27]. A recent paper suggested that depending on the disease states, age, and cell source, the colony formation capability of ECFCs and the numbers are different. For instance, the cord blood vs. children (age 0–10-years), the ECFCs number were high (9 and 5), while in the case of adults with middle aged or aged subjects, the level of ECFCs significantly declines up to 0.2 normalized to 10^7 MNCs [27]. It is presumed that in patients with concomitant diseases diabetes mellites or other, the quantity and quality of EPCs decreases up to zero colony formation [37].

Taken together, the origin of ECFCs origin is not defined and further studies are warranted to investigate its origin and *in vivo* presence.

EPCs Characterization *In Vivo*

So far, it has been considered a problem in the flow of research that the phenotype and function of EPC had to be discussed in terms of cultured phenotype "EPCs *ex vivo*". From a biological point of view, *the cells that differentiate into vascular endothelial cells in the living body should be defined as EPCs*. However, as is inevitable in biological research development, several discussions have concluded EPC biology based on research studies of cells that differentiate into ECs in culture *ex vivo*. We need to consider if these discussions for EPCs *ex vivo* are ultimately aimed at the cell biology of "EPCs *in vivo.*" In this regard, we discuss EPC biology based on the origin *in vivo*. Especially a majority of initial phase research utilized *CD34 positive* (CD34+) or *CD133 positive* (CD133+) cells in the human peripheral blood (PB) mononuclear cells and found its commitment into endothelial lineage cell *in vitro* and its integration into EC in new blood vessel formation *in vivo* [3, 13, 38-41]. These findings were supported by the irrefutable clinical pieces of evidence representing the CD34+ derived cells' incorporation into the human vasculature. Suzuki et al. reported significant EC replacement by BM-derived cells in acute radiation syndrome patients receiving G-CSF mobilized CD34+ cell transplantations [42]. The subsequent analysis of the aortas of these patients showed that approximately 25% of all ECs were replaced by ECs originating from the donors [42]. Jiang et al. demonstrated that 2% of ECs in the skin and gut from hematologic malignancy recipients who had undergone BM CD34+ cell transplantation was of donor origin [43]. Peters et al. determined that an average of 4.9% donor origin of blood vessels were detected in fluorescence *in situ* hybridization with sex chromosome-specific probes in the histological samples of various cancers after bone marrow transplantation with donor cells derived from individuals of the opposite sex [44].

However, several groups reported no contribution of transplanted BM-derived cells into the vasculature of implanted tumor grafts in host mice [45]. Others presented similar negative findings of EPC incorporation into the vasculature and contribution to blood vessel formation using various animal models, including a hindlimb ischemia model [46], a cytokine-induced angiogenesis model [47], a muscle injury model, and a non-injured cerebral nervous system model [48].

In this regard, it is noteworthy to mention that all reports stressing the failure of EPC incorporation and function studies-derived from non-human origin, utilizing mouse-based experiments primarily.

Tissue Resident EPC

A growing amount of evidence suggested the existence of tissue resident EPC along with circulatory EPC; additionally, in a lung injury model, tissue-resident pulmonary vascular endothelial cells (PVEC) significantly contributed to vascular repair and also highly expressed CD34, Flk-1/KDR, and c-kit more strongly and lesser CD133 cell surface marker in the proliferative phase rather than the nonproliferating PVEC in bone marrow chimera mice, indicating that bone marrow derived lung tissue-resident EPCs mainly contribute to pulmonary vascular repair after the onset of injury [49]. Another elegant EPC fate mapping experiment has clearly shown that PVEC proliferate *in situ* on the endothelial layer and that bone marrow derived EPCs are engrafted into the endothelial layer of lung microvessels at the active barrier repair phase by increasing the number of PVEC derived EC (CD45-/CD31+/BrdU+/ rtTA+) or bone marrow derived EPC (CD45-/CD31+/ eNOS+ /GFP+) by 22- or 121-fold, respectively [50]. Recently, Wakabayashi et al. identified CD157 as a marker of tissue-resident vascular endothelial stem cells (VESCs) in large arteries and veins of numerous mouse organs [51]. Single CD157+ VESCs form colonies *in vitro* and generate donor-derived portal veins, sinusoids, and central vein endothelial cells upon transplantation in the liver. In response to the injury, VESCs expand and regenerate entire vasculature structures, supporting the existence of an endothelial hierarchy within the blood vessels [51].

To sum up, the necessity of a new classification of EPC according to their source of origin, phenotype, function to delineate “true EPC” from “EPC like” cells is observed. The previous consensus statement on EPCs nomenclature needs to address these questions as it does not cover all of the aspects of "EPC" in the literature, which were described so far. A simplified classification may facilitate the appropriate clinical use of these cells.

Hematopoietic Cells Signal Cross-Talk on EPC Development

A seminal EPC study showed that the cocultures of CD34 depleted mononuclear cells with CD34+ cells significantly increased the proliferation rate and tube-like structure formation in fibronectin coated plates rather than CD34+ cells culturing along [13]. Subsequentially studies also implied that the crosstalk between hematopoietic cells with EPCs plays an important role in terms of EPC differentiation [22]. For example, T cells significantly accelerated primitive or small EPC-CFU, whereas macrophages and megakaryocytes solitarily promoted definitive or large EPC-CFU in *in vitro* assays in healthy human subjects, indicating that regenerative signals derived from myeloid or lymphoid cell subsets may cause vasculogenic or definitive EPC-CFU maturation [22]. However, over the last two decades, bone marrow mononuclear or purified CD34+ and CD133+ stem/cells transplantation clinical trials have been performed to cure various cardiovascular severe ischemic patients with modest results [52-54]. Perhaps, this may couple with qualitative and quantitative, along with crosstalk impairment of EPC with HSC subsets in patients with concomitant diseases, such as diabetes mellites, hypertension, atherosclerosis, hyperlipidemia, and along with risk-associated factors [55-59]. Moreover, the scarcity of EPC in peripheral blood, also mobilization obstacles in diabetes mellitus patients hamper to collect enough cells for the therapeutic application in clinical settings [55]. Following considerations, our group have developed a quality and quantity-controlled *ex vivo* culture (QQ-culture) system to educate mononuclear cells under vasculogenic signaling to increase regenerative cells for tissue regeneration. Notably, under vasculogenic conditioning, naïve PBMCs phenotype converted from pro-inflammatory (primitive EPC cells, M1 monocyte/macrophages (CD192+), Th1 (CD4+/INF-g+/IL4−), Natural killer cells (CD56+), and B cells (CD19+) etc. to anti-inflammatory polarized regenerative cells, such as definitive or vasculogenic EPC, M2ϕ (CD206+), T2 (CD4+/INF-g-/IL4+), regulatory T (CD4+/CD25+/FoxP3+) and regulatory B cells, and dendritic cells [23, 24, 60, 61] (Figure 2). This educated or regenerative conditioning induced PBMCs to represent as "*Regeneration-*

associated cells" (RACs) with several important properties of regeneration, such as immune modulatory, anti-inflammatory, and strong vasculogenic effects which were proved in *in vivo* experiments in different species [24, 61-63]. The aforementioned characteristics of RACs expand its clinical application ranges, such as cardiovascular ischemic diseases, including peripheral arterial diseases, myocardial impaction, and stroke etc.

The QQ culture technique was applied for peripheral blood derived MNCs to expand rare EPCs and showed that naïve proinflammatory PBMCs, the latter phenotype, was dramatically shifted to regenerative subsets, such as alternative activated M2, proangiogenic T cells along with definitive EPCs expansion. In EPC-CFA, vasculogenic conditioned MNCs dramatically increased dEPC-CFU formation with a high percentage of differentiation whereas fresh PBMCs formed a few colonies and most of them were in pEPC-CFU [24, 61]. In a hind limb ischemia (HLI) model of nude mice, we have evaluated RACs therapeutic efficacy vs Control, PBMNC, early EPC, and G-CSF mobilized CD34+ cells transplanted groups, respectively. The RAC transplanted groups started to accelerate ischemic leg blood flow perfusion and ischemia tissue recovery in contrast with the compared groups. The underlying mechanism of recovery by RAC may explain that RACs inhibit ischemia-induced inflammatory signals further leading to reparative process initiation in ischemic tissue being angiogenesis, arteriogenesis, myogenesis, while a natural course of ischemia usually includes tissue function loss like scar formation [24]. The other merits of RACs and RAC-derived extracellular vesicles (RAC-EVs) are that systemic and small cell dose transplantation can beneficially restore ischemic tissue functions via the preferential accumulation at the site of injury. In an acute myocardial ischemia model, we have shown that only small RACs dose ($1x10^5$ RACs transplanted via tail vein) markedly augmented the left ventricular hemodynamic functions by preferentially homing into the site of injury and developing an additional "biological bypass" to the ischemic host tissues [61, 64, 65]. Taken together, systemically transplanted RACs cells easily overcame lung and spleen barriers, preferentially accumulating into injured tissues to set in the motion of blood derived inflammatory cells phenotype transition into regenerative associated cells, such as EPCs, M2, Treg, angiogenic T and B cells in various ischemic organs [24, 61, 66, 67].

Conclusion: Unresolved Issues in EPC Biology and Future Perspectives

EPC biology has more questions rather than answers; there are several issues that need to be addressed in this field, such as:

1. Distinct delineating EPC surface markers need to be investigated using state of the art single cell genomics technology to define rare EPCs from circulation, but not in the culture. Notably, cultured cells are derivatives of circulating cells; however, although their differentiation traits may be ruled out by defined growth factors, the latter may not be corresponded or apart from real circulating EPCs along with their function.
2. It has been believed that EPCs originate from the bone marrow, and mobilize in response to ischemia, and home to the sites of vascular injury (9). However, recent findings demonstrated that circulating EPCs arise from an alternative niche in the vessel wall, but not from the bone marrow by using fluorescence *in situ* hybridization to detect X and Y chromosomes, and are supported by live cell imaging, flow cytometry, and immunofluorescence staining [34]. Similar findings were revealed by Li et al. wherein the structural integrity of the endothelium of the adult human heart during physiological conditions and following MI is maintained through the clonal proliferation of a subset of resident EPCs with minimal, if any, contribution from bone marrow cells using a single cell technology [63]. Another report claimed that the vessel derived CD34+ cells fraction is crucial for the endothelial repair of injured arteries [68]. To define the EPC contribution to vasculogenesis, sex mismatched bone-marrow transplanted large number of patients' recruitments of different ages, and fluorescence *in situ* hybridization to trace the EPCs origin is desired.
3. The crosstalk signals between EPCs and hematopoietic cells subsets, such as monocytes/macrophages, T cells, and B cells are crucial for EPCs differentiation and maintenance, which also need to be paid attention.
4. All of these notable findings need to be involved on EPCs classification for the development of an updated consensus, since the current consensus on EPCs nomenclature have not covered all of

EPCs by 1) source of origin, 2) *in vivo* presence, and 3) some misleading information, which we addressed in this chapter.

Disclosure

None.

References

[1] Asahara T. Murohara T. Sullivan A. Silver M. van der Zee R. Li T. Witzen-bichler B. Schatteman G. and Isner J. M. 1997. "Isolation of Putative Progenitor Endothelial Cells for Angiogenesis." *Science* 275: 964–7.

[2] Asahara T. Masuda H. Takahashi T. Kalka C. Pastore C. Silver M. Kearne M. Magner M. and Isner J. M. 1999. "Bone Marrow Origin of Endothelial Progenitor Cells Responsible for Postnatal Vasculogenesis in Physiological and Pathological Neovascularization." *Circulation Research* 85: 221–8.

[3] Shi Q. Rafii S. Wu M. H. Wijelath E. S. Yu C. Ishida A. Fujita Y. Kothari S. Mohle R. Sauvage L. R. Moore M. A. Storb R. F. and Hammond W. P. 1998. "Evidence for Circulating Bone Marrow-Derived Endothelial Cells." *Blood* 92: 362–7.

[4] Medina Reinhold J. Barber Chad L. Sabatier Florence, Dignat-George Francoise, Melero-Martin Juan M. Khosrotehrani Kiarash, Ohneda Osamu, Randi Anna M. Chan Jerry K. Y. Yamaguchi Teruhide, Van Hinsbergh Victor W. M. Yoder Mervin C. and Stitt Alan W. 2017. "Endothelial Progenitors: a Consensus Statement on Nomenclature." *Stem Cells Translational Medicine* 6: 1316–20.

[5] Hou Siyuan, Li Zongcheng, Zheng Xiaona, Gao Yun, Dong J. Ni Yanli, Wang Xiaobo, Li Yunqiao, Ding Xiaochen, Chang Zhilin, Li Shuaili, Hu Yuqiong, Fan Xiaoying, Hou Y. Wen L. Liu Bing, Tang Fuchou, and Lan Y. 2020. "Embryonic Endothelial Evolution Towards First Hematopoietic Stem Cells Revealed by Single-Cell Transcriptomic and Functional Analyses." *Cell Research* 30: 376–92.

[6] Jingyao Qiu, Karen K Hirschi. 2019. "Endothelial Cell Development and Its Application to Regenerative Medicine." *Circulation Research* 125.

[7] Michael J Chen, Tomomasa Yokomizo, Brandon M Zeigler, Elaine Dzierzak, Nancy A Speck. 2009. "Runx1 Is Required for the Endothelial to Haematopoietic Cell Transition but Not Thereafter." *Nature* 457.

[8] Gearges Lacaud, Valerie Kouskoff. 2017. "Hemangioblast, Hemogenic Endothelium, and Primitive versus Definitive Hematopoiesis." *Experimental Hematology* 49.

[9] Alexis S Bailey, Shuguang Jiang, Michael Afentoulis, Christina I Baumann, David A Schroeder, Susan B Olson, Melissa H Wong, William H Fleming. 2004. "Transplanted adult hematopoietic stems cells differentiate into functional endothelial cells. *Blood* 103(1).

[10] Case Jamie, Mead Laura E. Bessler Waylan K. Prater Daniel, White Hilary A. Saadatzadeh M. Reza, Bhavsar Janak R. Yoder Mervin C. Haneline Laura S. and Ingram David A. 2007. "Human CD34+AC133+VEGFR-2+ Cells Are Not Endothelial Progenitor Cells but Distinct, Primitive Hematopoietic Progenitors." *Experimental Hematology* 35: 1109–18.

[11] Mariusz Z Ratajczak, Janina Ratajczak, Magda Kucia. 2019. "Very Small Embryonic-Like Stem Cells (VSELs)." *Circulation Research* 124.

[12] Medina Reinhold J. Barber Chad L. Sabatier Florence, Dignat-George Francoise, Melero-Martin Juan M. Khosrotehrani Kiarash, Ohneda Osamu, Randi Anna M. Chan Jerry K. Y. Yamaguchi Teruhide, Van Hinsbergh Victor W. M. Yoder Mervin C. and Stitt Alan W. 2017. "Endothelial Progenitors: a Consensus Statement on Nomenclature." *Stem Cells Translational Medicine* 6: 1316–20.

[13] Asahara T. Murohara T. Sullivan A. Silver M. van der Zee R. Li T. Witzenbichler B. Schatteman G. and Isner J. M. et al. 1997 "Isolation of Putative Progenitor Endothelial Cells for Angiogenesis" *Science* 275: 964–7.

[14] Christoph Kalka, Haruchika Masuda, Tomono Takahashi, Wiltrud M. Kalka-Moll, Marcy Silver, Marianne Kearney, Tong Li, Jeffrey M. Isner, and Takayuki Asahara. "Transplantation of *Ex Vivo* Expanded Endothelial Progenitor Cells for Therapeutic Neovascularization." *Proceedings of the National Academy of Sciences of the United States of America*. 97.

[15] Hill Jonathan M. Zalos Gloria, Halcox Julian P J P. J. Schenke William H. Waclawiw Myron A. Quyyumi Arshed A. and Finkel Toren. 2003. "Circulating Endothelial Progenitor Cells, Vascular Function, and Cardiovascular Risk." *New England Journal of Medicine* 348: 593–600.

[16] Yoder Mervin C. Mead Laura E. Prater Daniel, Krier Theresa R. Mroueh Karim N. Li Fang, Krasich Rachel, Temm Constance J. Prchal Josef T. and Ingram David A. 2007. "Redefining Endothelial Progenitor Cells via Clonal Analysis and Hematopoietic Stem/Progenitor Cell Principals." *Blood* 109: 1801–9.

[17] Rohde Eva, Bartmann Christina, Schallmoser Katharina, Reinisch Andreas, Lanzer Gerhard, Linkesch Werner, Guelly Christian, and Strunk Dirk. 2007. "Immune Cells Mimic the Morphology of Endothelial Progenitor Colonies *In Vitro*." *Stem Cells* 25: 1746–52.

[18] Ingram David A. Mead Laura E. Tanaka Hiromi, Meade Virginia, Fenoglio Amy, Mortell Kelly, Pollok Karen, Ferkowicz Michael J. Gilley David, and Yoder Mervin C. 2004. "Identification of a Novel Hierarchy of Endothelial Progenitor Cells Using Human Peripheral and Umbilical Cord Blood." *Blood* 104: 2752–60.

[19] Hur Jin, Yoon Chang-Hwan, Kim Hyo-Soo, Choi Jin-Ho, Kang Hyun-Jae, Hwang Kyung-Kook, Oh Byung-Hee, Lee Myoung-Mook, and Park Young-Bae. 2004. "Characterization of Two Types of Endothelial Progenitor Cells and Their Different Contributions to Neovasculogenesis." *Arteriosclerosis, Thrombosis, and Vascular Biology* 24: 288–93.

[20] Timmermans Frank, Van Hauwermeiren Filip, De Smedt Magda, Raedt Robrecht, Plasschaert Frank, De Buyzere Marc L. Gillebert Thierry C. Plum Jean, and Vandekerckhove Bart. 2007. "Endothelial Outgrowth Cells Are Not Derived from

CD133+ Cells or CD45+ Hematopoietic Precursors." *Arteriosclerosis, Thrombosis, and Vascular Biology* 27: 1572–9.

[21] Fadini Gian Paolo, Losordo Douglas, and Dimmeler Stefanie. 2012. "Critical Re-Evaluation of Endothelial Progenitor Cell Phenotypes for Therapeutic and Diagnostic Use." *Circulation Research* 110: 624–37.

[22] Kwon Sang-Mo, Lee Jun-Hee, Lee Sang-Hun, Jung Seok-Yun, Kim Da-Yeon, Kang Song-Hwa, Yoo So-Young, Hong Jong-Kyu, Park Ji-Hye, Kim Jung-Hee, Kim Sung-Wook, Kim Yeon-Ju, Lee Sun-Jin, Kim Hwi-Gon, and Asahara Takayuki. 2014. "Cross Talk with Hematopoietic Cells Regulates the Endothelial Progenitor Cell Differentiation of CD34 Positive Cells." *PLOS ONE* 9: e106310.

[23] Masuda Haruchika, Alev Cantas, Akimaru Hiroshi, Ito Rie, Shizuno Tomoko, Kobori Michiru, Horii Miki, Ishihara Toshiya, Isobe Kazuya, Isozaki Mitsuhiro, Itoh Johbu, Itoh Yoshiko, Okada Yoshinori, McIntyre Brendan A. S. Kato Shunichi, and Asahara Takayuki. 2011. "Methodological Development of a Clonogenic Assay to Determine Endothelial Progenitor Cell Potential." *Circulation Research* 109: 20–37.

[24] Masuda H. Tanaka R. Fujimura S. Ishikawa M. Akimaru H. Shizuno T. Sato A. Okada Y. Iida Y. Itoh J. Itoh Y. Kamiguchi H. Kawamoto A. and Asahara T. 2014. "Vasculogenic Conditioning of Peripheral Blood Mononuclear Cells Prom-otes Endothelial Progenitor Cell Expansion and Phenotype Transition of Anti-Inflammatory Macrophage and T Lymphocyte to Cells with Regenerative Potential." *Journal of the American Heart Association* 3.

[25] Rossi Elisa, Poirault-Chassac Sonia, Bieche Ivan, Chocron Richard, Schnitzler Anne, Lokajczyk Anna, Bourdoncle Pierre, Dizier Blandine, Bacha Nour C. Gendron Nicolas, Blandinieres Adeline, Guerin Coralie L. Gaussem Pascale, and Smadja David M. 2019. "Human Endothelial Colony Forming Cells Express Intracellular CD133 That Modulates Their Vasculogenic Properties." *Stem Cell Reviews and Reports* 15: 590–600.

[26] Tasev Dimitar, Konijnenberg Lara S. F. Amado-Azevedo Joana, van Wijhe Michiel H. Koolwijk Pieter, and van Hinsbergh Victor W. M. 2016. "CD34 Expression Modulates Tube-Forming Capacity and Barrier Properties of Peripheral Blood-Derived Endothelial Colony-Forming Cells (ECFCs)." *Angiogenesis* 19: 325–38.

[27] Smadja David M. Melero-Martin Juan M. Eikenboom Jeroen, Bowman Mackenzie, Sabatier Florence, and Randi Anna M. 2019. "Standardization of Methods to Quantify and Culture Endothelial Colony-Forming Cells Derived from Peripheral Blood: Position Paper from the International Society on Thrombosis and Haemostasis SSC." *Journal of Thrombosis and Haemostasis: JTH* 17: 1190–4.

[28] Colombo Elena, Calcaterra Francesca, Cappelletti Monica, Mavilio Domenico, and Della Bella Silvia. 2013. "Comparison of Fibronectin and Collagen in Supporting the Isolation and Expansion of Endothelial Progenitor Cells from Human Adult Peripheral Blood." *PLOS ONE* 8: e66734.

[29] Wijelath Errol S. Rahman Salman, Murray Jacqueline, Patel Yatin, Savidge Geoffrey, and Sobel Michael. 2004. "Fibronectin Promotes VEGF-Induced CD34 Cell Differentiation into Endothelial Cells." *Journal of Vascular Surgery* 39: 655–60.

[30] Mannerström B. Paananen R. O. Abu-Shahba A. G. Moilanen J. Seppänen-Kaijansinkko R. and Kaur S. "Extracellular Small Non-Coding RNA Contaminants in Fetal Bovine Serum and Serum-Free Media". *Sci. Rep.:* 2019 9: 1–11.

[31] Wei Zhiyun, Batagov Arsen O. Carter David R. F. and Krichevsky Anna M.. 2016. "Fetal Bovine Serum RNA Interferes with the Cell Culture Derived Extracellular RNA". *Sci. Rep.*: 31175. *Scientific Reports* 6: 31175.

[32] Aswad Hala, Jalabert Audrey, and Rome Sophie. 2016. "Depleting Extracellular Vesicles from Fetal Bovine Serum Alters Proliferation and Differentiation of Skeletal Muscle Cells *In Vitro*." *BMC Biotechnology* 16: 32.

[33] Lin Y. Weisdorf D. J. Solovey A. and Hebbel R. P. 2000. "Origins of Circulating Endothelial Cells and Endothelial Outgrowth from Blood." *Journal of Clinical Investigation* 105: 71–7.

[34] Fujisawa Takeshi, Tura-Ceide Olga, Hunter Amanda, Mitchell Andrew, Vesey Alex, Medine Claire, Gallogly Susan, Hadoke Patrick W. F. Keith Charlotte, Sproul Anne, Roddie Huw, McQuaker Grant, Wilmut Ian, Mills Nicholas L. and Brittan Mairi. 2019. "Endothelial Progenitor Cells Do Not Originate from the Bone Marrow." *Circulation* 140: 1524–6.

[35] Ingram David A. Mead Laura E. Tanaka Hiromi, Meade Virginia, Fenoglio Amy, Mortell Kelly, Pollok Karen, Ferkowicz Michael J. Gilley David, and Yoder Mervin C. 2004. "Identification of a Novel Hierarchy of Endothelial Progenitor Cells Using Human Peripheral and Umbilical Cord Blood." *Blood* 104: 2752–60.

[36] Yi L. Daniel J. W. Anna S. and Robert P. H. 2000. "Origins of Circulating Endothelial Cells and Endothelial Outgrowth from Blood" *The Journal of Clinical Investigation* 105(1): 71–7.

[37] Pyšná Anna, Bém Robert, Němcová Andrea, Fejtarová Vladimíra, Jirkovská Alexandra, Hazdrová Jitka, Jude Edward B. and Dubský Michal. 2019. "Endothelial Progenitor Cells Biology in Diabetes Mellitus and Peripheral Arterial Disease and Their Therapeutic Potential." *Stem Cell Reviews and Reports* 15: 157–65.

[38] U M Gehling, S Ergün, U Schumacher, C Wagener, K Pantel, M Otte, G Schuch, P Schafhausen, T Mende, N Kilic, K Kluge, B Schäfer, D K Hossfeld, W Fiedler. "*In Vitro* Differentiation of Endothelial Cells from AC133-Positive Progenitor Cells." *Blood* 95.

[39] M Peichev, A J Naiyer, D Pereira, Z Zhu, W J Lane, M Williams, M C Oz, D J Hicklin, L Witte, M A Moore, S Rafii. 2000. "Expression of VEGFR-2 and AC133 by circulating human CD34(+) cells identifies a population of functional endothelial precursors." *Blood* 95.

[40] Toyoaki Murohara, Hisao Ikeda, Junli Duan, Satoshi Shintani, Ken-ichiro Sasaki, Hiroyuki Eguchi, Ichiro Onitsuka, Kazuo Matsui, and Tsutomu Imaizumi. 2000. "Transplanted cord blood-derived endothelial precursor cells augment postnatal neovascularization." *Journal of Clinical Investigation* 105.

[41] Erik B. Friedrich, Katrin Walenta, John Scharlau, Georg Nickenig, and Nikos Werner. 2006. "CD34-/CD133+/VEGFR-2+ Endothelial Progenitor Cell Subpopulation with Potent Vasoregenerative Capacities." *Circulation Research* 98.

[42] Toru Suzuki, Masamichi Nishida, Satory Futami, Keiko Fukio, Toshihiro Amaki, Kenishi Aizawa, et al. 2003. "Neoendothelialization After Peripheral Blood Stem

Cell Transplantation in Humans: A Case Report of a Tokaimura Nuclear Accident Victim. " *Cardiovasc Res.* 58(2).

[43] Shuguang Jiang, Luke Walker, Michael Afentoulis, Daniel A. Anderson, Linda Jauron-Mills, Christopher L. Corless, and William H. Fleming. 2004. "Transplanted Human Bone Marrow Contributes to Vascular Endothelium. " *Proceedings of the National Academy of Sciences of the United States of America.* 101(48).

[44] Brock A Peters, Luis A Diaz Jr, Kornelia Polyak, Leslie Meszler, Kathy Romans, Eva C Guinan, Joseph H Antin, David Myerson, Stanley R Hamilton, Bert Vogelstein, Kenneth W Kinzler & Christoph Lengauer. 2005. "Contribution of Bone Marrow-Derived Endothelial Cells to Human Tumor Vasculature." *Nature Medicine* 11.

[45] Michele De Palma, Mary Anna Venneri, Cristina Roca & Luigi Naldini. 2003. "Targeting Exogenous Genes to Tumor Angiogenesis by Transplantation of Genetically Modified Hematopoietic Stem Cells." *Nature Medicine* 9.

[46] Tibor Ziegelhoeffer, Borja Fernandez, Sawa Kostin, Matthias Heil, Robert Voswinckel, Armin Helisch, and Wolfgang Schaper. 2004. "Bone Marrow-Derived Cells Do Not Incorporate into the Adult Growing Vasculature." *Circulation Research* 94.

[47] Iiro Rajantie, Maritta Ilmonen, Agne Alminaite, Ugur Ozerdem, Kari Alitalo, Petri Salven. 2004. "Adult Bone Marrow-Derived Cells Recruited during Angiogenesis Comprise Precursors for Periendothelial Vascular Mural Cells." *Blood* 104.

[48] Francesco Galimi, Robert G. Summers, Henriette van Praag, Inder M. Verma, Fred H. Gage. 2005. "A role for bone marrow-derived cells in the vasculature of non-injured CNS." *Blood* 105.

[49] Kawasaki Takeshi, Nishiwaki Tetsu, Sekine Ayumi, Nishimura Rintaro, Suda Rika, Urushibara Takashi, Suzuki Toshio, Takayanagi Shin, Terada Jiro, Sakao Seiichiro, and Tatsumi Koichiro. 2015. "Vascular Repair by Tissue-Resident Endothelial Progenitor Cells in Endotoxin-Induced Lung Injury." *American Journal of Respiratory Cell and Molecular Biology* 53: 500–12.

[50] Mao Sun-Zhong, Ye Xiaobing, Liu Gang, Song Dongmei, and Liu Shu Fang. 2015. "Resident Endothelial Cells and Endothelial Progenitor Cells Restore Endothelial Barrier Function After Inflammatory Lung Injury." *Arteriosclerosis, Thrombosis, and Vascular Biology* 35: 1635–44.

[51] Wakabayashi Taku, Naito Hisamichi, Suehiro Jun-Ichi, Lin Yang, Kawaji Hideya, Iba Tomohiro, Kouno Tsukasa, Ishikawa-Kato Sachi, Furuno Masaaki, Takara Kazuhiro, Muramatsu Fumitaka, Weizhen Jia, Kidoya Hiroyasu, Ishihara Katsuhiko, Hayashizaki Yoshihide, Nishida Kohji, Yoder Mervin C. and Takakura Nobuyuki. 2018. "CD157 Marks Tissue-Resident Endothelial Stem Cells with Homeostatic and Regenerative Properties." *Cell Stem Cell* 22: 384–397.e6.

[52] Hirsch Alexander, Nijveldt Robin, van der Vleuten Pieter A. Tijssen Jan G P G. P. van der Giessen Willem J. Tio René A. Waltenberger Johannes, ten Berg Jurrien M. Doevendans Pieter A. Aengevaeren Wim R. M. Zwaginga Jaap Jan, Biemond Bart J. van Rossum Albert C. Piek Jan J. Zijlstra Felix, and HEBE Investigators. 2011. "Intracoronary Infusion of Mononuclear Cells from Bone Marrow or Peripheral Blood Compared with Standard Therapy in Patients after Acute Myocardial

Infarction Treated by Primary Percutaneous Coronary Intervention: Results of the Randomized Controlled HEBE Trial." *European Heart Journal* 32: 1736–47.

[53] Losordo Douglas W. Henry Timothy D. Davidson Charles, Sup Lee Joon, Costa Marco A. Bass Theodore, Mendelsohn Farrell, Fortuin F. David, Pepine Carl J. Traverse Jay H. Amrani David, Ewenstein Bruce M. Riedel Norbert, Story Kenneth, Barker Kerry, Povsic Thomas J. Harrington Robert A. Schatz Richard A. and ACT34-CMI Investigators. 2011. "Intramyocardial, Autologous CD34+ Cell Therapy for Refractory Angina." *Circulation Research* 109: 428–36.

[54] Losordo Douglas W. Kibbe Melina R. Mendelsohn Farrell, Marston William, Driver Vickie R. Sharafuddin Melhem, Teodorescu Victoria, Wiechmann Bret N. Thompson Charles, Kraiss Larry, Carman Teresa, Dohad Suhail, Huang Paul, Junge Candice E. Story Kenneth, Weistroffer Tara, Thorne Tina M. Millay Meredith, Runyon John Paul, Schainfeld Robert, and Autologous CD34+ Cell Therapy for Critical Limb Ischemia Investigators. 2012. "A Randomized, Controlled Pilot Study of Autologous CD34+ Cell Therapy for Critical Limb Ischemia." *Circulation. Cardiovascular Interventions* 5: 821–30.

[55] Fadini Gian Paolo, Albiero Mattia, Vigili de Kreutzenberg Saula Vd. Boscaro Elisa, Cappellari Roberta, Marescotti Mariacristina, Poncina Nicol, Agostini Carlo, and Avogaro Angelo. 2013. "Diabetes Impairs Stem Cell and Proangiogenic Cell Mobilization in Humans." *Diabetes Care* 36: 943–9.

[56] Rigato Mauro, Monami Matteo, and Fadini Gian Paolo. 2017. "Autologous Cell Therapy for Peripheral Arterial Disease: Systematic Review and Meta-Analysis of Randomized, Nonrandomized, and Noncontrolled Studies." *Circulation Research* 120: 1326–40.

[57] Puls Miriam, Schroeter Marco R. Steier Jasmin, Stijohann Lena, Hasenfuss Gerd, Konstantinides Stavros, and Schäfer Katrin. 2011. "Effect of Smoking Cessation on the Number and Adhesive Properties of Early Outgrowth Endothelial Progenitor Cells." *International Journal of Cardiology* 152: 61–9.

[58] Teraa Martin, Sprengers Ralf W. Schutgens Roger E. G. Slaper-Cortenbach Ineke C. M. van der Graaf Yolanda, Algra Ale, van der Tweel Ingeborg, Doevendans Pieter A. Mali Willem P. Th M. Moll Frans L. and Verhaar Marianne C. 2015. "Effect of Repetitive Intra-Arterial Infusion of Bone Marrow Mononuclear Cells in Patients with No-Option Limb Ischemia: the Randomized, Double-Blind, Placebo-Controlled Rejuvenating Endothelial Progenitor Cells via Transcutaneous Intra-Arterial Supplementation (JUVENTAS) Trial." *Circulation* 131: 851–60.

[59] Fadini Gian Paolo, Miorin Marta, Facco Monica, Bonamico Sondra, Baesso Ilenia, Grego Franco, Menegolo Mirko, de Kreutzenberg Saula Vigili, Tiengo Antonio, Agostini Carlo, and Avogaro Angelo. 2005. "Circulating Endothelial Progenitor Cells Are Reduced in Peripheral Vascular Complications of Type 2 Diabetes Mellitus." *Journal of the American College of Cardiology* 45: 1449–57.

[60] Masuda Haruchika, Iwasaki Hiroto, Kawamoto Atsuhiko, Akimaru Hiroshi, Ishikawa Masakazu, Ii Masaaki, Shizuno Tomoko, Sato Atsuko, Ito Rie, Horii Miki, Ishida Hideyuki, Kato Shunichi, and Asahara Takayuki. 2012. "Development of Serum-Free Quality and Quantity Control Culture of Colony-Forming Endothelial Progenitor Cell for Vasculogenesis." *Stem Cells Translational Medicine* 1: 160–71.

[61] Salybekov Amankeldi A. Kawaguchi Akira T. Masuda Haruchika, Vorateera Kosit, Okada Chisa, and Asahara Takayuki. 2018. "Regeneration-Associated Cells Improve Recovery from Myocardial Infarction through Enhanced Vasculogenesis, Anti-Inflammation, and Cardiomyogenesis." *PLOS ONE* 13: e0203244.

[62] Salybekov Amankeldi A. Masuda Haruchika, Miyazaki Kozo, Sheng Yin, Sato Atsuko, Shizuno Tomoko, Iida Yumi, Okada Yoshinori, and Asahara Takayuki. 2019. "Dipeptidyl dipeptidase-4 Inhibitor Recovered Ischemia through an Increase in Vasculogenic Endothelial Progenitor Cells and Regeneration-Associated Cells in Diet-Induced Obese Mice." *PLOS ONE* 14: e0205477.

[63] Tanaka Rica, Vaynrub Max, Masuda Haruchika, Ito Rie, Kobori Michiru, Miyasaka Muneo, Mizuno Hiroshi, Warren Stephen M. and Asahara Takayuki. 2013. "Quality-Control Culture System Restores Diabetic Endothelial Progenitor Cell Vasculogenesis and Accelerates Wound Closure." *Diabetes* 62: 3207–17.

[64] Salybekov Amankeldi A. Kunikeyev Aidyn D. Kobayashi Shuzo, and Asahara Takayuki. 2021. "Latest Advances in Endothelial Progenitor Cell-Derived Extracellular Vesicles Translation to the Clinic." *Frontiers in Cardiovascular Medicine* 8: 734562.

[65] Salybekov Amankeldi A. Salybekova Ainur, Sheng Yin, Shinozaki Yoshiko, Yokoyama Keiko, Kobayashi Shuzo, and Asahara Takayuki. 2021. "Extracellular Vesicles Derived from Regeneration Associated Cells Preserve Heart Function after Ischemia-Induced Injury." *Frontiers in Cardiovascular Medicine* 8: 754254.

[66] Ohtake Takayasu, Kobayashi Shuzo, Slavin Shimon, Mochida Yasuhiro, Ishioka Kunihiro, Moriya Hidekazu, Hidaka Sumi, Matsuura Ryo, Sumida Maki, Katagiri Daisuke, Noiri Eisei, Okada Kayoko, Mizuno Hiroshi, and Tanaka Rica. 2018. "Human Peripheral Blood Mononuclear Cells Incubated in Vasculogenic Conditioning Medium Dramatically Improve Ischemia/Reperfusion Acute Kidney Injury in Mice." *Cell Transplantation* 27: 520–30.

[67] Nakayama Taira, Nagata Eiichiro, Masuda Haruchika, Asahara Takayuki, and Takizawa Shunya. 2019. "Regeneration-Associated Cell Transplantation Contributes to Tissue Recovery in Mice with Acute Ischemic Stroke." *PLOS ONE* 14: e0210198.

[68] Liujun Jiang, Ting Chen, Shasha Sun, Ruilin Wang, Jiacheng Deng, Lingxia Lyu, Hong Wu, Mei Yang, Xiangyuan Pu, Luping Du, Qishan Chen, Yanhua Hu, Xiaosheng Hu, Yijiang Zhou, Qingbo Xu, and Li Zhang. 2021. "Nonbone Marrow CD34+ Cells are Crucial for Endothelial Repair of Injured Artery." *Circulation Research.* 129: e146-65.

Section II: EPC in Cardiovascular Diseases

Chapter 2

Diagnostic and Prognostic Potential of EPCs in Cardiovascular Diseases

Mehdi Hassanpour*
Shonan Research Institute of Innovative Medicine,
Shonan Kamakura General Hospital, Kamakura, Japan

Abstract

Recent scientific reports have proposed that the impairment of EPC is strongly associated with the evolution of CVDs. The quantity and quality of EPCs are supposed to reflect the vascular repair capacity. Dysfunctional EPC could be the first and probably reversible exhaustion clue of vascular regeneration mechanisms causing the emergence of endothelial impairment and vasculature damage in CVDs patients. Routine markers merely correlate with end stage-tissue injuries and there is a critical need for the detection of early stage of heart disease. EPCs quantification associate with the vascular network function and bring a clinical advantage over routine CVDs biomarkers. The present chapter highlights the prognostic role of circulating EPCs as a novel predictor of CVDs in some heart-related disorders.

Keywords: endothelial progenitor cells, cardiovascular disease, prognostic biomarker

* Corresponding Author's Email: hasanpourme@gmail.com.

In: Endothelial Progenitor Cells in Health and Disease
Editors: Amankeldi A. Salybekov, Shuzo Kobayashi and Takayuki Asahara
ISBN: 978-1-68507-794-5

Introduction

According to Dr. Thomas Sydenham, 17th century, "A man is as old as his arteries". This valuable quote demonstrates the focus of scientists on the cardiovascular system for decades, leads scientists to investigate cardio-vascular biology and vasculature senescence, and to highlight its studies on the associated mechanisms.

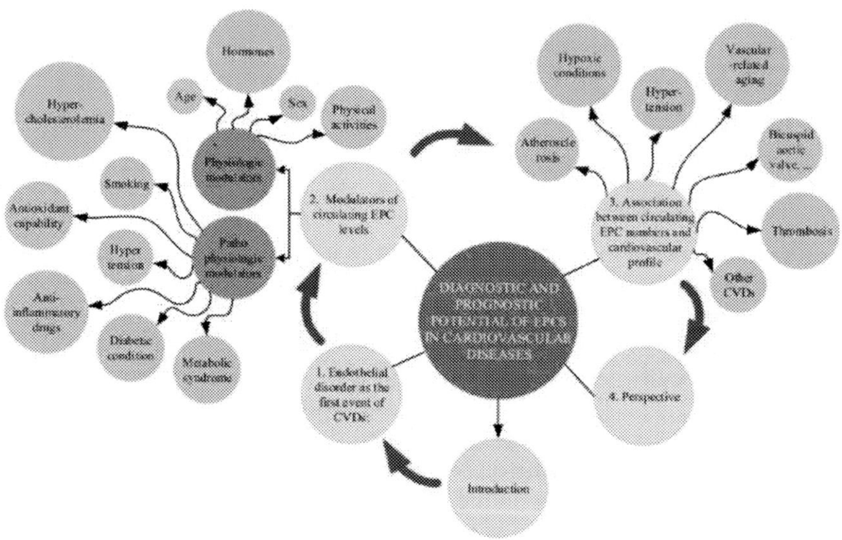

Figure 1. The graphical abstract of chapter.

According to WHO stratification, cardiovascular diseases (CVDs) are heterogeneous circulatory disorders, such as hypertensive, ischemic, and inflammatory heart diseases. Based on WHO statistics, approximately one third of global deaths are attributed to CVDs [1]. This significant fraction of mortality is avoidable with a precise early-stage diagnosis and subsequent proper treatment. The present chapter presents an overview of EPCs application as a biomarker for the early-stage detection of CVDs. The concept map of chapter is brought in Figure 1. Recently, cardiovascular studies have concentrated on endothelium network disorder and the underlying cellular-molecular mechanisms. Moreover, it is alleged that endothelium difficulties make up the initial pathophysiological complaint related to all CVDs. The gathering of endothelial cell (EC) injuries followed by an imbalance between death and the reparation process, symbolizes the beginning of endothelial malfunction. *In vivo* and *in vitro* experiments on endothelium biology have resulted in potential innovations in endothelium-related complications. Especially, one of the resolutions to tackle the onset of the endothelium-associated disorder is the comprehensive understanding of the biology of stem/progenitor cells, such as EPCs [2].

As mentioned in previous chapters, circulating EPCs are BM-derived blood mononuclear cells that have the capacity to proliferate, migrate, and differentiate into functional ECs [1]. Accumulated evidences have elucidated that EPCs not only provide a safe and feasible strategy for the treatment of CVDs, but are also considered as a biomarker for coronary and peripheral artery disease. Scientific literature has documented that the numbers and effectiveness of EPCs are decreases in numerous clinical disorders, such as diabetes [3, 4], hypertension [5], heart failure [6], and stroke [7, 8]. It has been reported that the quantity of peripheral EPC is decreased and EPC efficacy is weakened in both children [9] and adult patients with CVDs [10]. However, this result is controversial with AMI and refractory angina, demonstrating the increase in EPC levels in these patients [11, 12]. Importantly, the level of circulating EPCs further declined in the advanced stages of atherosclerosis in coronary [13], carotid [14], and atherosclerotic sites [15]. Furthermore, studies have shown that the relationships between severity of the atherosclerotic lesion and EPC levels, suggesting that low EPC levels present a biomarker of systemic atherosclerotic development [16]. Besides, circulating EPC levels are considerably decreased in refractory hypertension compared to healthy individuals [17]. In this respect, it is worth noting that hypertension accelerates EPC senescence in both experimental and hypertensive patients, supposing it to be related to telomerase inactivation [18, 19]. Also, hypertension-induced EPC aging affects vasculature remodeling [20]. Due to the controversy in this regard, the clear correlation between hypertension and the number of EPCs is not elucidated yet [21]. Valgimigli et al. reported that heart failure mobilizes EPC, with a rise and depression in the early and advanced stages, respectively [22]. The mobilization of EPCs is a response of a bone marrow niche to severe endothelial dysfunctionality during the early phases of heart failure [23]. Heart failure with a preserved ejection fraction (EF) is a progressively common status and is problematic to diagnose. Recently, a scientific report has shown that heart failure patients with both preserved and reduced EF have decreased circulating EPC numbers and increased the inflammatory reaction and N-terminal pro-BNP levels, compared to healthy subjects [24]. Moreover, Schwartzenberg et al. demonstrated that CD34/CD133 positive EPCs, but not the CD34/KDR positive or the CD133/KDR positive phenotypes, is prognostic of the upcoming adverse CVD outcomes [25].

Endothelial Disorder as the First Event of CVDs: EPCs as a Cellular Biomarker

The endothelium network has key functions as a guardian and principal sensor of physiochemical modifications in the circulation. Endothelium malfunction is a term for a shift from an intact endothelium to an impaired endothelium with proinflammatory characteristics. Notably, endothelium difficulties are the earliest pathological conditions for CVDs [26]. The endothelial disorder could be evaluated by invasive/non-invasive procedures. Nonetheless, these functional approaches provide shreds of evidence on the pathophysiological mechanism of dysfunction. As mentioned in the previous chapters, EPCs, not only provide facts about the endothelial cell homeostasis, but also present capable predictors, diagnostic, and prognostic biomarkers of CVDs. Although, EPCs barely exist in the peripheral blood in physiologic conditions, an increase in the EPCs level is typically observed in vascular damages and regeneration. Therefore, the presence of EPCs in the peripheral blood possibly will serve as a diagnostic or prognostic parameter of endothelial damage and regeneration rate. Actually, higher EPCs numbers indicate a greater regeneration and angiogenesis potency and the reduction of atherosclerosis progression and hypoxic endothelium injuries [26-28]. Additionally, it has been shown that diminished EPC levels accompany metabolic syndrome, which is one major risk factor for CVDs [29].

Modulators of Circulating EPC Levels

Physiological Modulators

The number of circulating EPCs in the physiologic condition is less than 0.01% of PBMNCs; nonetheless, numerous elements and situations could affect its levels and functionality [30]. As previously pointed out, the deficiencies in the mobilization, migration, recruitment, and utility of EPCs into endothelium networks occur in CVDs. Several endogenous and exogenous players modulate the circulating numbers and the functions of EPCs, and as negative and positive endogenous elements. With this in mind, for instance, endogenous factors, such as gender and pregnancy [31] and exogenous factors, such as lifestyle interventions (e.g. Mediterranean diet, exercise, and no smoking), hormonal agents, and drugs (e.g. statins) have been suggested as the potential factors to increase the EPC numbers and functionalities [32].

Estrogen

Estrogen has been alleged as a potent inducer of NO synthesis and eNOS motivation. Additionally, estrogen diminishes the level of eNOS inhibitor, named endogenous asymmetric dimethylarginine (ADMA) [33]. Regarding the effects of sex on the EPC levels, Fadini et al. have documented that estradiol acts as the biological inducer of EPC number, leading to higher EPC levels in women than men [31]. Also, pregnancy, leads to improvements in the circulating levels of EPC [34, 35]. This low number of EPCs may account for the fact of higher risk of CVDs risk in men.

Physical Activities

Physical activities induce NO production. It has been found that the number of circulating EPCs increases considerably after physical exercise for 28 days. Hypothetically, physical exercise causes NO production and NO production increases EPC levels both in the bone marrow and peripheral bloodstream [36].

Pathological Modulators

Scientific reports declare that patients with CVDs risk factors, including age, gender, smoking behaviors, hypertension, hyperglycemia, and hyperlipidemia decrease the level and functionality of EPCs [37].

It has been well-known that anti-inflammatory drugs, such as statin superfamily, as a member of HMG-CoA reductase inhibitors, have a direct correlation with the EPC number and functionality [38]. The statins upregulate PI3K/Akt pathway, leading to enhance the mobilization and function of EPCs [39]. Additionally, it has been well-documented that ACE inhibitors and peroxisome PPAR-γ agonists modify the EPC number and functionality, even though the underlying mechanisms are poorly understood [40]. However, persuasive documents suggest that the sustained exposure of the bone marrow source to chronic pro-inflammatory conditions regulate the EPC niche exhaustion. In such a situation, a small fraction of immature EPCs may be released into the bloodstream [66].

In the senescence process, there is an imbalance in the antioxidant capability because of the increase in free radicals and the unavailability of antioxidant agents that eventually caused diminished EPCs mobilization capability. Thus, both decreased clonogenic and migration capacity of EPC to VEGF factor in aged individuals seems logical [41]. For further validation, it has been noted that the survival, migration and proliferation potency, and overall functionality of the EPCs are reduced in aged individuals [42].

Smoking

Smoking is another risk factor causing endothelial dysfunctionality. The greater level of oxidative stress affects the mobilization and survival rate of EPC in smoking individuals compared to healthy individuals [43]. Besides, oxidative stress plays a key role in EPC mobilization from BM and functionality. Reactive oxygen species (ROS) has direct cytotoxicity effects on the vasculature network. The production of superoxide decreased EPC numbers and weakens the EPC function.

Hypertension

Hypertension is also considered by vasculature dysfunction and decreased NO production. In the early stage of hypertension, endothelial impairment could stimulate factors of EPCs mobilization as a remedial mechanism. In the late stages of hypertension and the beginning of oxidative stress and inflammation process, controversial effects start, i.e. decrease the number and functionality of EPCs [44, 45]. In hypertensive individuals, EPC aging is speeded and telomerase activity is reduced, causing vasculature remodeling [20]. EPCs impairment induces flawed endothelial repairment and dysfunctional angiogenesis, which induces the formation of atherosclerotic plaques [46]. In a study of refractory hypertensive patients, the circulating EPC levels were decreased significantly comparing with the healthy subjects via the downregulation of the CXCR4/JAK2/SIRT5 signaling pathway [17, 47]. Angiotensin II hastens the EPCs aging rate via oxidative stress [48]. Scientific reports have shown that the ramipril factor improves the number and functionality of EPCs [49]. Moreover, in another study, angiotensin II receptor antagonist therapy, including olmesartan/irbesartan, increases the EPCs quantity meaningfully after 4-week exposure [50].

Metabolic Syndrome

Metabolic syndrome contains a group of irregularities, including increased insulin resistance, hypertension, hyperglycemia, abdomen fat accumulation, and dyslipidemia, which increase the risk of CVDs, stroke, and type 2 diabetes [51]. Regarding the association between metabolic syndrome and EPC level, Westerweel et al. illustrated that the circulating CD34/KDR positive EPC numbers were decreased by approximately 40% in overweight individuals with metabolic syndrome compared to normal individuals [52]. Moreover, it has been documented that individuals with metabolic syndrome without CVDs show a decreased functionality of EPC (such as mobilization, migration, clonogenicity, and so forth) compared to healthy individuals [53]. These studies propose that EPCs impairment appears in metabolic syndrome prior to the development of CVDs. Notably, it has been shown that induced oxidative DNA damage, diminished telomerase function, and telomere length (as indications of the increased aging process) in EPCs of CVDs subjects with metabolic syndrome than subjects without metabolic syndrome [54]. Furthermore, the levels and functionality of EPC are decreased in the hepatic exhibition of metabolic syndrome, nonalcoholic fatty liver disease than subjects without nonalcoholic fatty liver disease [55]. These findings recommend that EPC modifications in the peripheral blood in metabolic syndrome could be one of the strategies to elucidate the progress of CVDs risk in metabolic syndrome conditions. For further support, Berezin et al. introduced EPC dysfunction as a biological marker of CVD risk in obese patients [56].

In diabetic conditions, the quality and quantity of circulating EPCs are decreased. Scientific evidence has illustrated that the proliferation potency of obtained EPCs from diabetic patients has reduced significantly compared with healthy subjects in both type 1 and type 2 diabetes [57, 58]. Treatment with antidiabetic agents, such as insulin, improves EPCs levels significantly in diabetic patients [59]. Insulin induces NO availability; however, insulin resistance decreases the NO production, produces a great amount of ROS, and downregulates PI3K/Akt, leading to a decrease in the reparation capacity and impaired mobilization [60, 61]. Also, Berezin et al. concluded that insulin-resistance is an additional factor, which participates in the decrease of circulating EPC levels in non-diabetic heart failure subjects [60].

Hypercholesterolemia

Hypercholesterolemia has an important correlation with vascular dysho-meostasis. It has been well-illustrated that the EPC levels are decreased considerably in hypercholesterolemic individuals. Besides, the number of EPCs has an inverse relationship with LDL-cholesterol [62]. However, HDL-cholesterol controls the quantity and quality of EPC by increasing eNOS and inhibiting apoptosis [63]. Moreover, Balistreri et al. reported that endocrine disorders, such as hyperparathyroidism and hypothyroidism, could change EPC properties [64]. Recently, it has been well elucidated that pharmacotherapies considerably affect the EPC numbers and properties and exert their anti-inflammatory and antioxidant effects. Lee et al. have reported that there is a considerable relationship between CVD drug therapies (i.e. antihypertension agents, cholesterol-lowering medicines, and antidiabetic drugs) and the increase of EPC levels and bio-functionality in clinical trials [65].

Association between Circulating EPC Numbers and Cardiovascular Profile

As mentioned, a strict relationship exists between the EPC circulating levels and cardiovascular risk profile. This may be of clinical relevance, and possible new recommendations and preventive CVD measures may arise as a result. Clinical trial studies carried out on CVDs patients propose that the EPC served as a novel biomarker. The circulating EPC levels have been introdused as a substitute marker for vasculature endothelium function because of the significant relationship between the number of EPC and flow-mediated brachial-artery reactivity and a decreased framingham risk factor score [66]. The investigations on EPCs shed new light on understanding the pathomechanism of both CVDs and atherosclerosis [67]. In addition, they found that *in vitro* EPC senescence reflects the risk profile of the donor's subjects. Thus, the authors suggested that EPCs might be considered to be an optimal biomarker for vascular function and cardiovascular risk [68]. Moreover, Berezin et al. have shown that EPCs dysfunction prognosticate the CVD possibility in the general population, patients with developed CVD, and metabolic disease [69]. Notably, EPCs obtained from individuals with CVDs have demonstrated a weakened migration and proliferation potency in subjects with risk factors of CVDs [70].

Also, our team has studied a notable investigation regarding the EPC levels in AMI. Salybekov et al. clarified that the total EPC count and their functionalities are inversely associated with glycated albumin and the mean amplitude of glycemic excursion (MAGE), which propose that hyperglycemia and the associated risk factors could decrease the EPC levels in AMI subjects compared to healthy subjects [71]. In support of this finding, it is worth noting that infarcted conditions deteriorate the intracellular antioxidant capacity. The accumulation of glycated end-products and LDL-cholesterol along with weakened antioxidant capacity induces mitochondrial DNA destruction and telomere shortening, promoting EPC aging. Notably, it has been shown that pathologic ischemic situations induce EPC generation in the bone marrow niche. However, these EPCs are not able to enter the peripheral bloodstream, parallel to the decreased EPCs mobilization response [72]. In other words, EPC proliferation is also increased; however, the maturation of EPCs into functional ECs is impaired. In line with this notion, it has been reported that EPC numbers reached their peak in the bloodstream at day 7 post-ischemia in AMI conditions. Also, Prof. Asahara's lab illustrated that, according to ROC curve analysis, EPC levels/mL in the bloodstream are independent, highly accurate, and predictive indicators of cardiac vessel injuries in the early phase of AMI. This observation is authorized by the inverse relationship of EPCs and cardiovascular injuries. Overall, herein, we clearly demonstrate the ability of EPCs to be used as a biomarker of heart vessel-lesions in the early phase of myocardial infarction. On a more general note, it could be said that the EPC count significantly decreased in the peripheral bloodstream after 3 days of AMI. Moreover, it suggests that the circulating EPCs correlated with the number of cardiac arteries injuries. In adittion, larger sample-sized studies are warranted to confirm the ability of EPCs and $CD8^+$ cells as the potential biomarkers of cardiac vessels of myocardial injuries, respectively, for the diagnosis and prognosis of AMI. The abnormalities in the circulating EPC levels and function have been observed in numerous studies on different CVDs [73]. In order to substantiate this role of EPCs, several pathological cardiovascular conditions are discussed in the following paragraphs.

Hypoxic Conditions

Studies showed that the EPC levels are increased considerably for a short-term after AMI onset and reached the highest level on the 7th day [74]. It has been well documented that the CD34 positive/CD45 negative EPC number increase in hypoxic conditions, such as AMI and acute coronary syndrome [75]. Hypoxic conditions initiate the synthesis of HIF-1α, causing the induction of transcription of VEGF, SDF-1α, and MCP-1, which energetically recruit EPCs from the bone marrow niche to the bloodstream and subsequently guide them to the hypoxic site. Besides, the indigenous status of the bone marrow has a central function in EPC mobilization. The cytokines of G-CSF, MMP-9, VEGF, SDF-1α, eNOS, and NO stimulate the mobilization process by interfering with the interaction between EPC and the other BM-derived stromal cells, allowing the EPCs to be released from the bone marrow through the endothelial sinusoid and entering the blood circulation. The process is the initial phase of EPCs mobilization from the bone marrow [76].

Atherosclerosis

The blood EPC count is suggested as an alternative marker for the risk of CVDs [77]. The main underlying mechanism of CVD is atherosclerosis [78]. Scientific reports have documented that hyperlipidemia causes lower EPC levels; additionally, vascular inflammatory reactions are an autonomous indicator for endothelium disorder and the advent of atherosclerosis. Recently, scientific reports declared that decreased EPC counts predict atherosclerosis development in an independent form, which supports a key function of vascular regeneration in CVDs. Communally, the improvement of dyslipidemia in subjects with CVDs is associated with a significant increase of EPC counts and enhances the risk of CVDs [79]. On the other hand, hypercholesterolemia is the major event initiating atherosclerosis, which induces the disruption of vascular endothelium integrity. In settings of endothelial damage, EPCs are mobilized from BM into circulation and are home to sites of vascular injury, where they aid endothelial regeneration and, subsequently, the regression of atherosclerosis. The researchers unanimously agree with Padfield et al. that the CD34 positive/CD45 negative EPC level reflects the incidence rate of atherosclerotic conditions and correlate with the number of atheromatous plaque lesions [80].

Thrombosis

Thrombosis is one of the major risk factors of CVDs, and exerts undesirable effects on vascular stem cells. In response to venous thrombosis, EPCs are mobilized from the bone marrow to the bloodstream in order to participate in endothelial regeneration. Erkek et al. studied the relationship between the EPC levels and thrombosis in paroxysmal nocturnal hemoglobinuria (PNH) patients and aplastic anemia patients. They showed that EPC numbers have a significant difference among patients with and without thrombosis [81], which was confirmed in thrombotic Behçet's syndrome [82]. In clinical settings, Lev et al. have reported that the EPC number was significantly reduced in the stent thrombosis group compared to the healthy group. Also, they showed that individuals suffering from late coronary stent thrombosis exhibited a decreased circulating EPC count and weakened functionalities of EPCs [83]. Besides, Bradbury et al. reported that low EPC numbers are significantly related with venous thrombosis. They declared that the D-dimer levels were conversely associated with a low EPC count [84]. Nevertheless, temporary increases in the EPC numbers may appear to promote revascularization during acute ischemia and thrombosis. In a convincing study, it has been shown that microRNA-483-3p is upregulated in the EPCs of deep vein thrombosis patients, impairing the EPCs functionalities through a serum response factor. For further support, they illustrated that the administration of EPCs transfected with microRNA-483-3p suppressor into the experimental thrombosis model of rats upgraded the resolution of the thrombotic site [85]. Nosaka et al. convincingly proposed that the levels of intra-thrombotic EPC above 20 may predict a thrombus age defined in the neighborhood of 7–14 days and acts as a tool for accurate thrombus age estimation [86]. If EPC quantification is confirmed to predict venous thrombosis recurrence, it will recommend a novel prognostic and diagnostic biomarker to provide a decision-making approach for the early treatment of patients. Additional larger trials are desirable to authorize the predictive value of EPC quantification for the recurrence of venous thrombosis.

Hypertension

Hypertension is one of the main risk factors for CVDs. Recently, the scientific society has inclined on the possible association between hypertension and EPCs. Cumulative evidence has documented a great relationship between the EPC counts and hypertension [87, 88] that is supported in the refractory hypertension context [89]. Vasa's group highlighted that the hypertensive context leads to decrease in the EPC levels and their functionalities, such as migration potency [90]. In this regard, it is mentioned that essential hypertensive conditions lead to the elevation of markers of renal vein and inflammation reactions in essential hypertensive individuals and are correlated with increased inflamed ECs and diminished EPC counts [91]. Consistently, MacEneaney and coworkers showed the clonogenicity of EPCs decreased significantly in prehypertensive individuals (130 mmHg < systolic blood pressure < 139 mmHg) upon comparison with the normotensive group [92]. However, the underlying mechanism of defective effects of hypertension on EPCs is poorly understood. A higher secretion of cytokines and inflamed ECs weakens the EPC regeneration capability in essential hypertensive conditions. This condition could intensify the vascular injury and increase the hypertension-associated mortality rates in essential hypertensive subjects. At the same time, according to Braitsch and colleagues, hypertension-related cardiac fibrosis involves a specific sub-phenotype of EPC, named TCF-21 positive cells. It is worth noting that TCF-21 is expressed during embryonic heart evolution and promotes cardiac fibroblast development and inhibits smooth muscle cells differentiation of epicardium-derived cells [93]. Pirro et al. have documented that never-treated hypertensive patients showed reduced EPC count and homeobox A9 expression in comparison with normotensive subjects [94]. They concluded that hypertensive conditions downregulate the expression level of homeobox A9 in circulating EPCs, which may have a predictive role in low EPC levels of hypertensive patients. For further support, Rossig et al. have shown that homeobox A9-suppressed mice have decreased EPC numbers compared to physiologic mice, while homeobox A9 expression in peripheral blood MNCs elevates the EPC yield [95]. Also, it has been reported that hypertensive rats showed decreased EPC levels, which is related to reduced telomerase activity enhanced senescence of EPCs [20, 96]. Mechanistically, angiotensin II incites the beginning of EPC senescence thorough the induction of oxidative stress, NADPH oxidase activation, decreased telomerase activity, LDL oxidation, and the suppression of the Akt pathway [97]. From another viewpoint, in addition to causation, it has been hypothesized that a high bloodstream provokes EPC death both in hypertensive experimental models and hypertensive patients [20, 98], impairing the quantity and quality of EPCs. Likewise, antihypertensive agents increase the EPC numbers and recover EPC functionality [99]. Based on this viewpoint, it was found that ramipril therapy, as an antihypertensive agent, is related to a remarkable increase in homeobox A9 expression, leading to a rise in the EPC count [94]. Also, Umemura et al. evaluated the effects of renin–angiotensin system inhibitors, as antihypertensive drugs on EPCs levels, showing a significant correlation between antihypertensive therapy and increase in the EPCs count [100].

Vascular-Related Aging

With advancing age, all cell types are subject to internal alterations that ultimately cause the cell to meet an irreversible proliferation arrest phase, named senescence. This section is aimed to describe the detective role of EPCs in aging, as a CVD risk factor. Previous studies validated that the self-renewal potency and levels of stem/progenitors is completely influenced by age-related alterations [101]. Recently, we well displayed that the proliferative capacity and clonogenicity of EPCs is influenced by senescence in human, canine, and murine-derived EPCs [42]. For supporting our findings, Povsic and coworkers declared that the number of circulating EPCs diminished by aging through decreasing expression levels of Tie-2 and VEGFR genes [102]. Also, it has been documented that the number and migration/adhesion potency of EPCs were meaningfully declined with the advance of age in experimental models and clinical studies [103]. Moreover, the EPC levels decrease conversely with aging in patients with CVDs [104]. Vasa et al. analyzed the age-related reduction of circulating EPCs in aged healthy and AMI subjects [105]. However, the question whether the EPCs correlate with the aging of individuals has remained unclear. Mandraffino et al. designed an investigation to assess the potency of CD34 positive EPCs to anticipate the long-term viability in octogenarians. They declared that the subjects with lower baseline of CD34 positive EPCs showed a higher mortality rate after 7 years of monitoring. Furthermore, the CD34 positive EPCs count was remarkably greater in subjects of older age at demise or were still alive at the end of the study. They recommended that the greater the EPC levels, the greater the odds of survival [106]. Aging abolishes the hemostasis of proteomic and genomic machineries. For example, aging induces histone demodification, such as H2AX phosphorylation, H3K56 acetylation, and H3K79 methylation, causing telomere shortening [107]. EPC aging stimulated by telomere shortening possibly leads to quantificational weakening of EPCs and decrease of the vascular regeneration capability in the aging endothelium. Remarkably, the upregulation of the human telomerase reverse transcriptase (hTERT) gene in circulating angiogenic cells conserves the telomerase activity, delays the cell aging process, and augments the EPC regenerative properties in an experimental murine model of ischemic hind limb [108]. Increased oxidative stress and oxidized-LDL, as hallmarks of senescence have been related with EPCs senescence, which decrease their level and function impairing. Additionally, a correlation between the oxidative DNA damage and decreased telomere length of EPCs derived from coronary artery disease patients has been observed [109]. According to Balistreri et al. it could be assumed that the combined evaluation of the RDW levels hs-CRP and circulating EPCs present the best prognosticator of vascular aging independently, providing a suitable biomarker for the prediction of age-related diseases, such as sporadic ascending aorta aneurysm. They displayed that age risk factor significantly decreased the EPCs count in old subjects compared to young subjects, suggesting that old healthy individuals have a reduced number of circulating EPCs and consequently reduced reparative capabilities of the cardiovascular system. However, upcoming investigations are definitely needed for authenticating the relevance of these findings [104].

Bicuspid Aortic Valve, Aortic Valve Regurgitation and Aneurysm

Several studies demonstrated that the individuals suffering from bicuspid aortic valve and valvular difficulties display low levels of EPCs with weakened functionalities. In consistence with this outcome, Shimoni et al. clarified that the EPCs levels are reduced in patients with aortic regurgitation compared to normal individuals with the same risk factors without valve involvement. Notably, this outcome was obvious in subjects with different aortic regurgitation etiologies [110]. In patients with aortic regurgitation, the EPC number is inversely associated with the left ventricular thickness, male gender, and left ventricular end-systolic diameter. Additionally, the EPCs are supposed to have a central function in aneurysm pathology, neointima synthesis, and angiogenic process in rabbit experimental models [111].

Other CVDs

Despite the above-mentioned cardiovascular conditions, the predictive function of EPCs has been explored in other cardiac pathophysiologies and peripheral vascular disorders. In this regard, Chan et al. revealed that the EPC (CD133/KDR positive type) levels were meaningfully elevated in PR interval elongation syndrome subjects [112]. Furthermore, it has been demonstrated that higher drug resistance to phosphodiesterase type 5 inhibitors is related to a higher rate of EC apoptosis in arterial erectile dysfunction, which is accompanied by higher circulating late EPCs numbers. Additionally, Rodrigo et al.

evaluated that the EPCs count is decreased in patients with sickle cell anemia, which increases the risk of CVD [113].

Conclusion

EPCs bring a clinical advantage over routine CVD biomarkers, including MB creatine kinase, cardiac troponin I, NT-pro-BNP, oxidized LDL, and C reactive protein. The quantification of the circulating EPC count and functionality associate with the vascular network function, while routine markers merely correlate with end-stage-tissue injuries or stress. The medical community is following new strategies to face the imposing challenge of CVD. Particularly, the latest innovations in the field of EPC biology and their potency to provide a prognostic clue for treatments of CVDs are causing investigators to focus their attention on EPC as a promising novel treatment with natural reparative capacity. Additionally, applying comprehensive machine learning-based methods, such as artificial intelligence-assisted predictive approaches, enable us to accurately check the cardiovascular system. A large body of evidence demonstrates that modifications in the level and functionalities of EPCs suggestively associated with CVDs. Such discoveries highlight the hypothesis that EPCs could be served as a potential diagnostic and prognostic factor regarding a better risk biomarker of the CVDs, although several aspects still remain to be elucidated. Firstly, it is obligatory to authenticate the validity of the actual data because of the lack of regulated approaches for the quantification of EPCs. A unique EPC characterization and exact description are indispensable and further investigations will be required to establish uniform principles for EPC identification, procedure, and approaches. This could elucidate the detailed biological functions of EPCs and authenticate their clinical applications as biomarkers or as a cell source for cell therapy. Taken together, the road is still difficult, and long and large clinical trials are essential for the comprehensive description of whether EPC impairment is a witness of the physiological progress of the CVDs. In one more general note, well-planned comprehensive clinical trials and monitoring of the quantity and quality of circulating EPCs as well as applying artificial intelligence-assisted predictive approaches are obligatory to decipher the true prognostic/diagnostic value of EPCs for CVDs patients.

References

[1] Noale M, Limongi F, Maggi S. Epidemiology of cardiovascular diseases in the elderly. *Frailty and Cardiovascular Diseases*. 2020: 29-38.

[2] Wang Y, Tissenbaum HA. Overlapping and distinct functions for a Caenorhabditis elegans SIR2 and DAF-16/FOXO. *Mechanisms of Ageing and Development.* 2006; 127(1): 48-56.

[3] Zhang J, Li Y, Li H, Zhu B, Wang L, Guo B, et al. GDF11 improves angiogenic function of EPCs in diabetic limb ischemia. *Diabetes*. 2018; 67(10): 2084-95.

[4] Fadini GP, Miorin M, Facco M, Bonamico S, Baesso I, Grego F, et al. Circulating endothelial progenitor cells are reduced in peripheral vascular complications of type 2 diabetes mellitus. *Journal of the American College of Cardiology*. 2005; 45(9): 1449-57.

[5] Zhu S, Deng S, Yang F, Zhang T, Afshartous D, Goldschmidt PJ, et al. Reduced Endothelial Progenitor Cells (EPCs) in Patients with Severe Hypertension. *Amer Heart Assoc*. 2010.

[6] Liu Z-L, Wu Z-S, Hu J-G, Yang Y-F, Chen Y, Gao H, et al. Correlation of serum levels of VEGF and SDF-1 with the number and function of circulating EPCs in children with cyanotic congenital heart disease. *Zhongguo dang dai er ke za zhi= Chinese Journal of Contemporary Pediatrics*. 2009; 11(4): 267-72.

[7] Krenning G, Dankers PY, Drouven JW, Waanders F, Franssen CF, van Luyn MJ, et al. Endothelial progenitor cell dysfunction in patients with progressive chronic kidney disease. *American Journal of Physiology-Renal Physiology*. 2009; 296(6): F1314-F22.

[8] Ozkok A, Yildiz A. Endothelial progenitor cells and kidney diseases. *Kidney and Blood Pressure Research*. 2018; 43(3): 701-18.

[9] Abdel-Salam M, Abd Elsalam R, Youssef N, Mamdouh F, Abdel-Salam T. Evaluation of endothelial progenitor cell (CD34) as a marker of cardiovascular risk in children on regular hemodialysis. *Saudi Journal of Kidney Diseases and Transplantation*. 2018; 29(4): 785.

[10] Kou F, Zhu C, Wan H, Xue F, Wang J, Xiang L, et al. Endothelial progenitor cells as the target for cardiovascular disease prediction, personalized prevention, and treatments: progressing beyond the state-of-the-art. *EPMA Journal*. 2020: 1-15.

[11] Shintani S, Murohara T, Ikeda H, Ueno T, Honma T, Katoh A, et al. Mobilization of endothelial progenitor cells in patients with acute myocardial infarction. *Circulation*. 2001; 103(23): 2776-9.

[12] Güven H, Shepherd RM, Bach RG, Capoccia BJ, Link DC. The number of endothelial progenitor cell colonies in the blood is increased in patients with angiographically significant coronary artery disease. *Journal of the American College of Cardiology*. 2006; 48(8): 1579-87.

[13] Fadini GP, Losordo D, Dimmeler S. Critical reevaluation of endothelial progenitor cell phenotypes for therapeutic and diagnostic use. *Circulation Research*. 2012; 110(4): 624-37.

[14] Lau K, Chan Y, Yiu K, Li S, Tam S, Lau C, et al. Burden of carotid atherosclerosis in patients with stroke: relationships with circulating endothelial progenitor cells and hypertension. *Journal of Human Hypertension*. 2007; 21(6): 445-51.

[15] Xiao Q, Kiechl S, Patel S, Oberhollenzer F, Weger S, Mayr A, et al. Endothelial progenitor cells, cardiovascular risk factors, cytokine levels and atherosclerosis–results from a large population-based study. *PloS one*. 2007; 2(10): e975.

[16] Liu P, Zhou B, Gu D, Zhang L, Han Z. Endothelial progenitor cell therapy in atherosclerosis: a double-edged sword? *Ageing Research Reviews*. 2009; 8(2): 83-93.

[17] Oliveras A, Soler M, Martinez-Estrada O, Vazquez S, Marco-Feliu D, Vila J, et al. Endothelial progenitor cells are reduced in refractory hypertension. *Journal of Human Hypertension*. 2008; 22(3): 183-90.

[18] Imanishi T, Kobayashi K, Hano T, Nishio I. Effect of estrogen on differentiation and senescence in endothelial progenitor cells derived from bone marrow in spontaneously hypertensive rats. *Hypertension Research*. 2005; 28(9): 763-72.

[19] Diller G-P, van Eijl S, Okonko DO, Howard LS, Ali O, Thum T, et al. Circulating endothelial progenitor cells in patients with Eisenmenger syndrome and idiopathic pulmonary arterial hypertension. *Circulation*. 2008; 117(23): 3020-30.

[20] Imanishi T, Moriwaki C, Hano T, Nishio I. Endothelial progenitor cell senescence is accelerated in both experimental hypertensive rats and patients with essential hypertension. *Journal of Hypertension*. 2005; 23(10): 1831-7.

[21] Boos C, Goon P, Lip G. Endothelial progenitor cells in the vascular pathophysiology of hypertension: arterial stiffness, ageing and more. *Journal of Human Hypertension*. 2006; 20(7): 475-7.

[22] Valgimigli M, Rigolin GM, Fucili A, Porta MD, Soukhomovskaia O, Malagutti P, et al. CD34+ and endothelial progenitor cells in patients with various degrees of congestive heart failure. *Circulation*. 2004; 110(10): 1209-12.

[23] Deng Y, Wang J, He G, Qu F, Zheng M. Mobilization of endothelial progenitor cell in patients with acute ischemic stroke. *Neurological Sciences*. 2018; 39(3): 437-43.

[24] Chiang C-H, Huang P-H, Leu H-B, Hsu C-Y, Wang K-F, Chen J-W, et al. Decreased circulating endothelial progenitor cell levels in patients with heart failure with preserved ejection fraction. *Cardiology*. 2013; 126(3): 191-201.

[25] Schwartzenberg S, Afek A, Charach G, Rubinstein A, Ben-Shoshan Y, Kissil S, et al. Comparative analysis of the predictive power of different endothelial progenitor cell phenotypes on cardiovascular outcome. *World Journal of Cardiology*. 2010; 2 (9): 299.

[26] Cahill PA, Redmond EM. Vascular endothelium–Gatekeeper of vessel health. *Atherosclerosis*. 2016; 248: 97-109.

[27] Critser PJ, Yoder MC. Endothelial colony forming cell role in neoangiogenesis and tissue repair. *Current Opinion in Organ Transplantation*. 2010; 15(1): 68.

[28] Madonna R, Novo G, Balistreri CR. Cellular and molecular basis of the imbalance between vascular damage and repair in ageing and age-related diseases: as biomarkers and targets for new treatments. *Mechanisms of Ageing and Development*. 2016; 159: 22-30.

[29] Devaraj S, Jialal I. Dysfunctional endothelial progenitor cells in metabolic syndrome. *Experimental Diabetes Research*. 2012; 2012.

[30] Huizer K, Mustafa DA, Spelt JC, Kros JM, Sacchetti A. Improving the characterization of endothelial progenitor cell subsets by an optimized FACS protocol. *PLoS One*. 2017; 12(9): e0184895.

[31] Fadini GP, de Kreutzenberg S, Albiero M, Coracina A, Pagnin E, Baesso I, et al. Gender differences in endothelial progenitor cells and cardiovascular risk profile: the role of female estrogens. *Arteriosclerosis, Thrombosis, and Vascular Biology*. 2008; 28(5): 997-1004.

[32] Hristov M, Weber C. Endothelial progenitor cells: characterization, pathophysiology, and possible clinical relevance. *Journal of Cellular and Molecular Medicine*. 2004; 8(4): 498-508.

[33] Davison S, Davis SR. New markers for cardiovascular disease risk in women: impact of endogenous estrogen status and exogenous postmenopausal hormone therapy. *The Journal of Clinical Endocrinology & Metabolism*. 2003; 88(6): 2470-8.

[34] Mallucci G, Beneventi F, Bergamaschi R, Bizzotto C, Cavagnoli C, De Maggio I, et al. Circulating endothelial progenitor cells during pregnancy in multiple sclerosis. *Neurological Sciences*. 2021; 42(4): 1443-51.

[35] Robb AO, Mills NL, Newby DE, Denison FC. Endothelial progenitor cells in pregnancy. *Reproduction*. 2007; 133(1): 1-9.

[36] Laufs U, Werner N, Link A, Endres M, Wassmann S, Jürgens K, et al. Physical training increases endothelial progenitor cells, inhibits neointima formation, and enhances angiogenesis. *Circulation*. 2004; 109(2): 220-6.

[37] Di Stefano R, Felice F, Feriani R, Balbarini A. Endothelial progenitor cells, cardiovascular risk factors and lifestyle modifications. *Internal and Emergency Medicine*. 2013; 8(1): 47-9.

[38] Briguori C, Quintavalle C, D'Alessio F, Donahue M, Roscigno G, De Micco F, et al. Impact of statin therapy intensity on endothelial progenitor cells after percutaneous coronary intervention in diabetic patients. The REMEDY-EPC late study. *International Journal of Cardiology*. 2017; 244: 112-8.

[39] Pirro M, Schillaci G, Romagno PF, Mannarino MR, Bagaglia F, Razzi R, et al. Influence of short-term rosuvastatin therapy on endothelial progenitor cells and endothelial function. *Journal of Cardiovascular Pharmacology and Therapeutics*. 2009; 14(1): 14-21.

[40] Tan Q, Zhang S, Li Y. Circulating endothelial progenitor cells were decreased in patients with metabolic syndrome. *Clinical Laboratory*. 2018; 64(10): 1679-83.

[41] Hoetzer GL, Van Guilder GP, Irmiger HM, Keith RS, Stauffer BL, DeSouza CA. Aging, exercise, and endothelial progenitor cell clonogenic and migratory capacity in men. *Journal of Applied Physiology*. 2007; 102(3): 847-52.

[42] Hassanpour M, Cheraghi O, Siavashi V, Rahbarghazi R, Nouri M. A reversal of age-dependent proliferative capacity of endothelial progenitor cells from different species origin in *in vitro* condition. *Journal of Cardiovascular and Thoracic Research*. 2016; 8(3): 102.

[43] Michaud SÉ, Dussault S, Haddad P, Groleau J, Rivard A. Circulating endothelial progenitor cells from healthy smokers exhibit impaired functional activities. *Atherosclerosis*. 2006; 187(2): 423-32.

[44] Tousoulis D, Andreou I, Antoniades C, Tentolouris C, Stefanadis C. Role of inflammation and oxidative stress in endothelial progenitor cell function and mobilization: therapeutic implications for cardiovascular diseases. *Atherosclerosis*. 2008; 201(2): 236-47.

[45] Saad MI, Abdelkhalek TM, Saleh MM, Kamel MA, Youssef M, Tawfik SH, et al. Insights into the molecular mechanisms of diabetes-induced endothelial dysfunction: focus on oxidative stress and endothelial progenitor cells. *Endocrine*. 2015; 50(3): 537-67.

[46] Kolluru GK, Bir SC, Kevil CG. Endothelial dysfunction and diabetes: effects on angiogenesis, vascular remodeling, and wound healing. *International Journal of Vascular Medicine*. 2012.

[47] Yu B-B, Zhi H, Zhang X-Y, Liang J-W, He J, Su C, et al. Mitochondrial dysfunction-mediated decline in angiogenic capacity of endothelial progenitor cells is associated with capillary rarefaction in patients with hypertension via down regulation of CXCR4/JAK2/SIRT5 signaling. *EBio Medicine*. 2019; 42: 64-75.

[48] Kobayashi K, Imanishi T, Akasaka T. Endothelial progenitor cell differentiation and senescence in an angiotensin II-infusion rat model. *Hypertension Research*. 2006; 29(6): 449-55.

[49] Min TQ, Zhu CJ, Xiang WX, Hui ZJ, Peng SY. Improvement in endothelial progenitor cells from peripheral blood by ramipril therapy in patients with stable coronary artery disease. *Cardiovascular Drugs and Therapy*. 2004; 18(3): 203-9.

[50] Bahlmann FH, de Groot K, Mueller O, Hertel B, Haller H, Fliser D. Stimulation of endothelial progenitor cells: a new putative therapeutic effect of angiotensin II receptor antagonists. *Hypertension*. 2005; 45(4): 526-9.

[51] Saklayen MG. The global epidemic of the metabolic syndrome. *Current Hypertension Reports*. 2018; 20(2): 1-8.

[52] Westerweel PE, Visseren FL, Hajer GR, Olijhoek JK, Hoefer IE, de Bree P, et al. Endothelial progenitor cell levels in obese men with the metabolic syndrome and the effect of simvastatin monotherapy vs. simvastatin/ezetimibe combination therapy. *European Heart Journal*. 2008; 29(22): 2808-17.

[53] Jialal I, Devaraj S, Singh U, Huet B. Decreased number and impaired functionality of endothelial progenitor cells in subjects with metabolic syndrome: implications for increased cardiovascular risk. *Atherosclerosis*. 2010; 211(1): 297-302.

[54] Satoh M, Ishikawa Y, Takahashi Y, Itoh T, Minami Y, Nakamura M. Association between oxidative DNA damage and telomere shortening in circulating endothelial progenitor cells obtained from metabolic syndrome patients with coronary artery disease. *Atherosclerosis*. 2008; 198(2): 347-53.

[55] Chiang C-H, Huang P-H, Chung F-P, Chen Z-Y, Leu H-B, Huang C-C, et al. Decreased circulating endothelial progenitor cell levels and function in patients with nonalcoholic fatty liver disease. *PloS one*. 2012; 7(2): e31799.

[56] Berezin AE. Endothelial progenitor cell dysfunction as a biomarker of cardio-vascular risk in obese patients. *ARC Journal of Diabetes and Endocrinology*. 2016; 2(2): 12-5.

[57] Longo M, Scappaticcio L, Bellastella G, Pernice V, Cirillo P, Maio A, et al. Alterations in the levels of circulating and endothelial progenitor cells levels in young adults with type 1 diabetes: a 2-year follow-up from the observational metro study. *Diabetes, Metabolic Syndrome and Obesity: Targets and Therapy*. 2020; 13: 777.

[58] Zhai L, Liu Y, Zhao W, Chen Q, Guo T, Wei W, et al. Aerobic and resistance training enhances endothelial progenitor cell function via upregulation of caveolin-1 in mice with type 2 diabetes. *Stem Cell Research & Therapy*. 2020; 11(1): 1-11.

[59] Kusuyama T, Omura T, Nishiya D, Enomoto S, Matsumoto R, Takeuchi K, et al. Effects of treatment for diabetes mellitus on circulating vascular progenitor cells. *Journal of Pharmacological Sciences*. 2006; 102(1): 96-102.

[60] Berezin AE, Kremzer AA. Relationship between circulating endothelial progenitor cells and insulin resistance in non-diabetic patients with ischemic chronic heart failure. *Diabetes & Metabolic Syndrome: Clinical Research & Reviews*. 2014; 8(3): 138-44.

[61] Kahn MB, Yuldasheva NY, Cubbon RM, Smith J, Rashid ST, Viswambharan H, et al. Insulin resistance impairs circulating angiogenic progenitor cell function and delays endothelial regeneration. *Diabetes*. 2011; 60(4): 1295-303.

[62] Chen JZ, Zhang FR, Tao QM, Wang XX, Zhu JH, Zhu JH. Number and activity of endothelial progenitor cells from peripheral blood in patients with hypercholest-erolaemia. *Clinical Science*. 2004; 107(3): 273-80.

[63] Noor R, Shuaib U, Wang CX, Todd K, Ghani U, Schwindt B, et al. High-density lipoprotein cholesterol regulates endothelial progenitor cells by increasing eNOS and preventing apoptosis. *Atherosclerosis*. 2007; 192(1): 92-9.

[64] Balistreri CR, Buffa S, Pisano C, Lio D, Ruvolo G, Mazzesi G. Are endothelial progenitor cells the real solution for cardiovascular diseases? Focus on controversies and perspectives. *BioMed Research International*. 2015; 2015.

[65] Qiu Y, Zhang C, Zhang G, Tao J. Endothelial progenitor cells in cardiovascular diseases. *Aging Medicine*. 2018; 1(2): 204-8.

[66] Schmidt-Lucke C, Rössig L, Fichtlscherer S, Vasa M, Britten M, Kämper U, et al. Reduced number of circulating endothelial progenitor cells predicts future cardio-vascular events: proof of concept for the clinical importance of endogenous vascular repair. *Circulation*. 2005; 111(22): 2981-7.

[67] Liu JH, Chen Y, Zhen Z, Yeung CK, Chan J, Chan HH, et al. Relation between endothelial progenitor cells and arterial stiffness in patients with psoriasis. *The Journal of Dermatology*. 2016; 43(8): 888-93.

[68] Hill JM, Zalos G, Halcox JP, Schenke WH, Waclawiw MA, Quyyumi AA, et al. Circulating endothelial progenitor cells, vascular function, and cardiovascular risk. *New England Journal of Medicine*. 2003; 348(7): 593-600.

[69] Berezin AE, Kremzer AA, Martovitskaya YV, Berezina TA, Gromenko EA. Pattern of endothelial progenitor cells and apoptotic endothelial cell-derived microparticles

in chronic heart failure patients with preserved and reduced left ventricular ejection fraction. *EBioMedicine*. 2016; 4: 86-94.

[70] Berezin A. Impaired phenotype of endothelial cell-derived microparticles: causality factor contributed the "vascular competence" in diabetes and metabolic syndrome. *Diabetes Res Treat Open Access*. 2016; 3: 133-6.

[71] Salybekov A, Sakai K, Natsumeda M, Vorateera K, Kobayashi S, Ikari Y, et al. *Peripheral Levels of EPCs, T Cells, and Macrophages' as Possible Predictive Biomarkers of Acute Myocardial Infarction.* Accessed from https://www.researchsquare.com/article/rs-107073/v1. 2020.

[72] Salybekov AA, Masuda H, Miyazaki K, Sheng Y, Sato A, Shizuno T, et al. Dipeptidyl dipeptidase-4 inhibitor recovered ischemia through an increase in vasculogenic endothelial progenitor cells and regeneration-associated cells in diet-induced obese mice. *Plos One*. 2019; 14(3): e0205477.

[73] Kröpfl JM. Circulating progenitor cells as predictor of mortality in cardiovascular disease: Could physical activity change the global outcome? *Atherosclerosis*. 2021.

[74] Morrone D, Felice F, Scatena C, De Martino A, Picoi M, Mancini N, et al. Role of circulating endothelial progenitor cells in the reparative mechanisms of stable ischemic myocardium. *International Journal of Cardiology*. 2018; 257: 243-6.

[75] Morishita T, Uzui H, Nakano A, Mitsuke Y, Geshi T, Ueda T, et al. Number of endothelial progenitor cells in peripheral artery disease as a marker of severity and association with pentraxin-3, malondialdehyde-modified low-density lipoprotein and membrane type-1 matrix metalloproteinase. *Journal of Atherosclerosis and Thrombosis*. 2012; 19(2): 149-58.

[76] Minhajat R, Nilasari D, Bakri S. The role of endothelial progenitor cell in cardiovascular disease risk factors. *Acta Medica Indonesiana*. 2015; 47(4).

[77] Berezin AE. Could be used an immune phenotypes of circulating endothelial progenitor cells as a biomarker of cardiovascular disease? *ARC Journal of Cardiology*. 2017; 3(1):9-12.

[78] Vergès B. Cardiovascular disease with type 1 diabetes: A review of epidemiological data and underlying mechanisms. *Diabetes & Metabolism*. 2020.

[79] Croce G, Passacquale G, Necozione S, Ferri C, Desideri G. Nonpharmacological treatment of hypercholesterolemia increases circulating endothelial progenitor cell population in adults. *Arteriosclerosis, Thrombosis, and Vascular Biology*. 2006; 26(5): e38-e9.

[80] Padfield GJ, Tura-Ceide O, Freyer E, Barclay GR, Turner M, Newby DE, et al. Endothelial progenitor cells, atheroma burden and clinical outcome in patients with coronary artery disease. *Heart*. 2013; 99(11): 791-8.

[81] Erkek ET, Nazligul E, Nalcaci M, Yenerel MN. Circulating endothelial progenitor cells and their relation to thrombosis in paroxysmal nocturnal hemoglobinuria and aplastic anemia. *Indian Journal of Hematology and Blood Transfusion*. 2021: 1-8.

[82] Bozkirli E, Keskek S, Kozanoglu I, Yucel A. High levels of endothelial progenitor cells can be associated with thrombosis in patients with Behçet's disease. *Clin Exp Rheumatol*. 2014; 32(4 Suppl 84): S49-53.

[83] Lev E, Leshem-Lev D, Harel N, Dvir D, Greenberg G, Assali A, et al. editors. Circulating endothelial progenitor cells in patients who underwent late coronary stent thrombosis. *European Heart Journal*; 2009; 31(21):2625-32

[84] Bradbury CA, Buckley T, Fletcher K, Rose P, Fitzmaurice D. Lower levels of circulating endothelial progenitor cells are associated with increased recurrence after unprovoked venous thrombosis. *Blood*. 2016; 128(22): 3805.

[85] Kong L, Hu N, Du X, Wang W, Chen H, Li W, et al. Upregulation of miR-483-3p contributes to endothelial progenitor cells dysfunction in deep vein thrombosis patients via SRF. *Journal of Translational Medicine*. 2016; 14(1): 1-14.

[86] Nosaka M, Ishida Y, Kimura A, Yamamoto H, Kato T, Kuninaka Y, et al. Detection of intrathrombotic endothelial progenitor cells and its application to thrombus age estimation in a murine deep vein thrombosis model. *International Journal of Legal Medicine*. 2017; 131(6): 1633-8.

[87] Ontiyuelo CM, Chiaradía DAR, Blanco I, Ceide OT, Pin AR, Herranz A, et al. Effects of endurance exercise training on circulating endothelial progenitor cells and endothelial microparticles in patients with pulmonary arterial hypertension. *Eur Respiratory Soc*, 2020.

[88] Shi L, Zhang Y, Lin Y, Cui X, Li J, Lin S. A13240 circulating endothelial cells and endothelial progenitor cells in relation to the severity of primary hypertension in children. *Journal of Hypertension*. 2018; 36: e219.

[89] Budzyń M, Gryszczyńka B, Boruczkowski M, Kaczmarek M, Begier-Krasińska B, Osińska A, et al. The potential role of circulating endothelial cells and endothelial progenitor cells in the prediction of left ventricular hypertrophy in hypertensive patients. *Frontiers in Physiology*. 2019; 10: 1005.

[90] Oktaviono YH, Hutomo SA, Luke K. The role of endothelial progenitor cells in coronary artery disease: basic molecular mechanisms and its clinical potentials. *The Indonesian Biomedical Journal*. 2021; 13(2): 106-13.

[91] Savoia C, Sada L, Zezza L, Pucci L, Lauri FM, Befani A, et al. Vascular inflammation and endothelial dysfunction in experimental hypertension. *International Journal of Hypertension*. 2011; 2011.

[92] MacEneaney OJ, DeSouza CA, Weil BR, Kushner EJ, Van Guilder GP, Mestek M, et al. Prehypertension and endothelial progenitor cell function. *Journal of Human Hypertension*. 2011; 25(1): 57-62.

[93] Braitsch CM, Kanisicak O, van Berlo JH, Molkentin JD, Yutzey KE. Differential expression of embryonic epicardial progenitor markers and localization of cardiac fibrosis in adult ischemic injury and hypertensive heart disease. *Journal of Molecular and Cellular Cardiology*. 2013; 65: 108-19.

[94] Pirro M, Schillaci G, Menecali C, Bagaglia F, Paltriccia R, Vaudo G, et al. Reduced number of circulating endothelial progenitors and HOXA9 expression in CD34+ cells of hypertensive patients. *Journal of Hypertension*. 2007; 25(10): 2093-9.

[95] Rössig L, Urbich C, Brühl T, Dernbach E, Heeschen C, Chavakis E, et al. Histone deacetylase activity is essential for the expression of HoxA9 and for endothelial commitment of progenitor cells. *Journal of Experimental Medicine*. 2005; 201(11): 1825-35.

[96] van Zonneveld A-J, Rabelink TJ. Endothelial progenitor cells: biology and therapeutic potential in hypertension. *Current Opinion in Nephrology and Hypertension.* 2006; 15(2): 167-72.

[97] Imanishi T, Hano T, Nishio I. Angiotensin II accelerates endothelial progenitor cell senescence through induction of oxidative stress. *Journal of Hypertension.* 2005; 23(1): 97-104.

[98] Huang P-H, Huang S-S, Chen Y-H, Lin C-P, Chiang K-H, Chen J-S, et al. Increased circulating CD31+/annexin V+ apoptotic microparticles and decreased circulating endothelial progenitor cell levels in hypertensive patients with microalbuminuria. *Journal of Hypertension.* 2010; 28(8): 1655-65.

[99] De Ciuceis C, Rossini C, Tincani A, Airò P, Scarsi M, Agabiti-Rosei C, et al. Effect of antihypertensive treatment with lercanidipine on endothelial progenitor cells and inflammation in patients with mild to moderate essential hypertension. *Blood Pressure.* 2016; 25(6): 337-43.

[100] Umemura T, Soga J, Hidaka T, Takemoto H, Nakamura S, Jitsuiki D, et al. Aging and hypertension are independent risk factors for reduced number of circulating endothelial progenitor cells. *American Journal of Hypertension.* 2008; 21(11): 1203-9.

[101] Josephson AM, Bradaschia-Correa V, Lee S, Leclerc K, Patel KS, Lopez EM, et al. Age-related inflammation triggers skeletal stem/progenitor cell dysfunction. *Proceedings of the National Academy of Sciences.* 2019; 116(14): 6995-7004.

[102] Povsic TJ, Sloane R, Pieper CF, Pearson MP, Peterson ED, Cohen HJ, et al. Endothelial progenitor cell levels predict future physical function: an exploratory analysis from the VA enhanced fitness study. *Journals of Gerontology Series A: Biomedical Sciences and Medical Sciences.* 2016; 71(3): 362-9.

[103] Yang J-X, Pan Y-Y, Wang X-X, Qiu Y-G, Mao W. Endothelial progenitor cells in age-related vascular remodeling. *Cell Transplantation.* 2018; 27(5): 786-95.

[104] Balistreri CR, Pisano C, Bertoldo F, Massoud R, Dolci S, Ruvolo G. Red Blood Cell distribution width, vascular aging biomarkers, and endothelial progenitor cells for predicting vascular aging and diagnosing/prognosing age-related degenerative arterial diseases. *Rejuvenation Research.* 2019; 22(5): 399-408.

[105] Scheubel RJ, Zorn H, Silber R-E, Kuss O, Morawietz H, Holtz J, et al. Age-dependent depression in circulating endothelial progenitor cells inpatients undergoing coronary artery bypass grafting. *Journal of the American College of Cardiology.* 2003; 42(12): 2073-80.

[106] Mandraffino G, Sardo MA, Riggio S, D'Ascola A, Alibrandi A, Saitta C, et al. Circulating progenitor cells and the elderly: a seven-year observational study. *Experimental Gerontology.* 2012; 47(5): 394-400.

[107] Pagiatakis C, Musolino E, Gornati R, Bernardini G, Papait R. Epigenetics of aging and disease: a brief overview. *Aging Clinical and Experimental Research.* 2021; 33(4): 737-45.

[108] Murasawa S, Llevadot J, Silver M, Isner JM, Losordo DW, Asahara T. Constitutive human telomerase reverse transcriptase expression enhances regenerative properties of endothelial progenitor cells. *Circulation.* 2002; 106(9): 1133-9.

[109] Tao J, Yang Z, Wang J-M, Wang L-C, Luo C, Tang A, et al. Shear stress increases Cu/Zn SOD activity and mRNA expression in human endothelial progenitor cells. *Journal of Human Hypertension*. 2007; 21(5): 353-8.

[110] Shimoni S, Bar I, Zilberman L, Goland S, Edri O, Gandelman G, et al. Circulating progenitor and apoptotic progenitor cells in patients with aortic regurgitation. *Circulation Journal*. 2013; 77(3): 764-71.

[111] Van Spyk EN, Chun KC, Samadzadeh KM, Peters JH, Lee ES. Increased levels of CD34+ cells are associated in patients with abdominal aortic aneurysms compared with patients with peripheral vascular disease. *Journal of Surgical Research*. 2013; 184(1): 638-43.

[112] Chan Y-H, Siu C-W, Yiu K-H, Yiu Y-F, Lau K-K, Lam T-H, et al. Prolongation of PR interval is associated with endothelial dysfunction and activation of vascular repair in high-risk cardiovascular patients. *Journal of Interventional Cardiac Electrophysiology*. 2013; 37(1): 55-61.

[113] Rodrigo M, Mendelsohn L, Bereal-Williams C, Hunter L, Dalby CK, McGowan V, et al. Circulating endothelial progenitor cells in adults with sickle cell disease. *Pulmonary Circulation*. 2013; 3(2): 448-9.

Chapter 3

Epidemiology of Peripheral Artery Disease

Takayasu Ohtake[1,2,3,*],
and Shuzo Kobayashi, MD, PhD[2,3]
[1]Regenerative Medicine,
Center for Cell Therapy and Regenerative Medicine,
Shonan Kamakura General Hospital, Kamakura, Japan
[2]Shonan Research Institute of Innovative Medicine,
Shonan Kamakura General Hospital, Kamakura, Japan
[3]Kidney and Transplant Center,
Shonan Kamakura General Hospital,
Kamakura, Japan

Abstract

Peripheral artery disease (PAD) is observed to be more common than previously estimated. PAD, frequently merging with coronary artery disease and/or cerebrovascular disease, constitutes polyvascular disease. In cases of CLTI (critical limb-threatening ischemia), the most severe devastating manifestation of PAD, limb and life salvage becomes a major concern because poor outcomes are reported. Revascularization therapy is an optimal and essential treatment for CLTI. However, more than half of CLTI patients could not be the candidate for revascularization, and these patients might inevitably wait for limb amputation or death. Revascularization therapy could rescue many severely ischemic limbs. However, the result has still not yet reached to an optimal level. End-stage renal disease (ESRD)/hemodialysis (HD) is strongly impacted due

* Corresponding Author's Email: ohtake@shonankamakura.or.jp.

In: Endothelial Progenitor Cells in Health and Disease
Editors: Amankeldi A. Salybekov, Shuzo Kobayashi and Takayuki Asahara
ISBN: 978-1-68507-794-5

to its prevalence and difficulty of treatment. ESRD patients have several non-traditional risk factors for atherosclerosis and they have to live with these multiple factors.

Regenerative therapy for CLTI will be precisely provided in another chapter. Here, we summarize the epidemiology of PAD/CLTI with special concern on the characteristic features in ESRD/HD patients.

Keywords: peripheral artery disease, critical limb-threatening ischemia, hemodialysis, revascularization, risk factor

Introduction

The arterial system from the iliac artery to the foot is the longest peripheral arterial structure in human body. The peripheral arteries to the lower limbs are composed of the common iliac artery, superficial femoral artery, popliteal artery, anterior and posterior tibial arteries, peroneal arteries, and dorsal and pedal arteries. In the atherosclerotic condition, any arteries mentioned above could be targeted for stenosis or occlusion, leading to limb ischemia. Peripheral arteries play an important role in the supplying of blood flow (oxygen and nutrients) to muscles in the lower limbs, which occupy more than 50% of the total body muscles. Lower limbs are essential for walking; additionally, a significant amount of oxygen is necessary for muscles in the lower limbs for walking. Therefore, the lower limbs would be particularly affected by ischemia due to the arterial stenosis or occlusion in the lower limbs.

Peripheral artery disease (PAD) refers to the atherosclerotic obstruction of the arteries of the lower extremities. Non-invasive measures, such as ankle brachial index (ABI) provided asymptomatic PAD is much more common than expected. The spreading of ABI as a screening test and ABI values < 0.9 as PAD definition unveiled the high prevalence of PAD in the world (>200 million patients in the world) [1]. Among the several clinical stages of PAD, critical limb threatening ischemia (CLTI) is the most severe life and limb-threatening manifestation of PAD, with clinical symptoms including resting pain or ischemic ulcers/gangrene in the lower extremities. Revascularization therapy, including endovascular therapy or bypass surgery is an optimal and essential treatment for CLTI. However, more than 50% of patients with CLTI could not be the candidate for revascularization therapy; additionally, these patients have no optional treatment to save their limbs and/or their lives, leading to limb amputation or death [2]. The discovery of circulating endothelial progenitor cells (EPCs) by Asahara et al. a landmark discovery in vascular medicine, provided a novel EPC-based cell therapy as a therapeutic approach in PAD/CLTI [3]. Recently, EPCs are used for not only intractable CLTI, but also for a variety of organ dysfunctions, including kidney disease, liver cirrhosis, and spinal injury [4-8]. Here, we summarize the recent epidemiological findings in patients with PAD/CLTI with special concern on the characteristic features in patients with end-stage renal disease (ESRD).

Epidemiology

A recent worldwide systematic review for PAD revealed that approximately 236 million individuals, aged 25 years and older had PAD in the world. The major risk factors were age, smoking, diabetes, hypertension, and dyslipidemia as in coronary artery disease or stroke [9]. Chronic kidney disease (CKD) is also an important independent risk factor for PAD/CLTI [10, 11]. The association of ABI < 0.9 with renal insufficiency was independent of potential confounders, such as age, diabetes, hypertension, coronary artery disease (CAD), stroke, and hypercholesterolemia [10]. A nationwide database in Japan including more than one million patients revealed that the prevalence of ESRD in patients with CLTI who underwent endovascular therapy (EVT) was significantly higher than that in patients with coronary artery disease (CAD), who underwent percutaneous coronary intervention (PCI) (6.39-times, $p < 0.01$) [12]. ESRD might more closely contribute to CLTI than CAD who needed PCI and be the most significant risk factor for PAD and progression to CLTI. A higher body mass index (BMI) was also significantly correlated with an increased risk of PAD [13]. A positive association between BMI and PAD was significantly stronger in patients with CLTI than those without CLTI.

PAD is the third most common clinical manifestation of atherosclerosis after coronary artery disease and stroke [1]. The Reduction of Atherothrombosis for Continued Health (REACH) Registry provided an international prevalence of patients with atherothrombosis [14]. The authors collected data on atherosclerosis risk factors from 67,888 patients with established arterial disease or 3 or more risk factors for atherothrombosis. Polyvascular disease, defined as having two or more vascular diseases, including coronary artery disease (CAD), cerebrovascular disease (CVD), and PAD, was shown in 15.9% of the total patients. PAD with CAD and/or CVD was shown in 7.5%

among the total patients. More than half of PAD patients have CAD and/or CVD in the REACH registry (Figure 1).

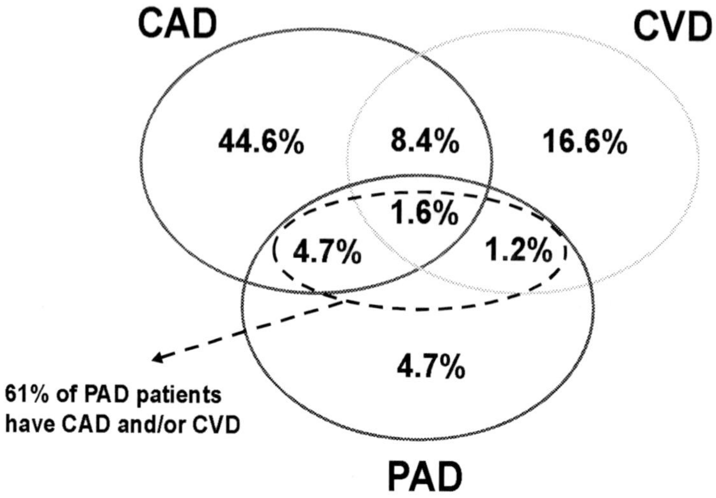

Figure 1. Prevalence of polyvascular disease in REACH Registry.
Abbreviations: CAD (coronary artery disease); CVD (cerebrovascular disease); PAD (peripheral artery disease); REACH (Reduction of Atherothrombosis for Continued Health).

A population based observational study revealed the long-term prognoses of PAD patients with different clinical stages. The 10-year all-cause mortality rate was 27% for cases with an ABI value more than 0.9 and no symptoms, 56% for asymptomatic PAD, 63% for intermittent claudication, and 75% for severe limb ischemia [15]. Even if the patients with PAD are asymptomatic, the cardiovascular event risk was significantly higher than that in patients without PAD. Cardiovascular events were the main cause of death (45%) in PAD patients. The Intersociety Consensus for the management of PAD estimated that 25% of patients with CLTI will die within 1 year and 30% will undergo limb amputation [16]. The 5-year mortality rate of patients with PAD is worse than that of breast cancer and Hodgkin's disease [17]. Because most patients with CLTI will eventually undergo some type of revascularization, it might be difficult to define the natural atheros of CLTI. However, a systematic review with meta-analysis for untreated CLTI revealed a rate of all-cause mortality of 22%, a rate of major amputation of 22%, and the rate of wound/ulcer worsening of 35% during a median follow-up of 12 months [18].

Characteristics of PAD in CKD Patients

ESRD is an independent risk factor for the development of PAD [19]. As in the general population, the traditional cardiovascular risk factors, including age, smoking, diabetes, hypertension, and dyslipidemia are associated with an increased risk of PAD. However, these risk factors cannot not fully explain the high prevalence of PAD in patients with ESRD. The onset and progression of PAD are associated with the characteristic factors in ESRD, i.e. uremic milieu, chronic microinflammation, malnutrition, immunodeficiency, higher BMI, and CKD mineral bone disorder (CKD-MBD) accompanied by accelerated vascular calcification (Figure 2) [20-25]. Malnutrition and chronic inflammation in uremic milieu form a vicious pathophysiological condition, i.e. malnutrition-inflammation-atherosclerosis (MIA) syndrome [26, 27], and causes accelerated progression of atherosclerosis, worsening the prognosis of dialysis patients with PAD. Immunodeficiency in uremia, accompanied by malnutrition, increases the susceptibility to wound infection, leading to an increased risk for major amputation of the lower limbs. Both malnutrition and wound infections are independent predictors of delayed wound healing [28]. Obese sarcopenia is recently shown to correlate with an increased risk of PAD in HD patients [29]. As these multiple non-traditional ESRD-characteristic risk factors add on to the traditional risk factors, the atherosclerotic process remarkably accelerates in dialysis patients. As shown in the REACH study, a high prevalence of polyvascular disease was shown in hemodialysis (HD) patients [23]. HD patients with PAD showed a significantly high prevalence of vascular complications including ischemic heart disease (IHD) and stroke compared with those without PAD. IHD was shown almost approximately 50% or more in prevalent HD patients with PAD regardless of the clinical severity of PAD. Notably, even though the stage of PAD was very mild (asymptomatic Fontaine classification I), almost half of the patients had IHD (Table 1) [23]. The characteristic features of PAD shown in HD patients are extensive vascular calcification and more distal peripheral vascular involvement. Vascular calcification is promoted from the non-dialytic earlier stages of CKD (Stage IIIb) [24], and accelerates after the initiation of HD [23]. The degree of vascular calcification in the arteries of the lower limbs was significantly correlated with the severity of PAD in HD patients [23].

It is to be noted that the prevalence of PAD is very high in ESRD patients, i.e. 24.3% at the time of HD initiation [30] and 16.5 ~ 41.4% in patients on maintenance HD [31, 32]. Further, 70% of incident HD patients with PAD were asymptomatic. However, a careful follow up is necessary because some cases rapidly develop CLTI without apparent preceding symptoms. The cumulative incident CLTI rate reaches up to 15% at 5 years after the initiation of HD [33]. In Japan, more than half of the CLTI patients who underwent revascularization are HD dependent [34-37]. Thus, ESRD/dialysis has a considerable impact on the onset and progression of PAD/CLTI.

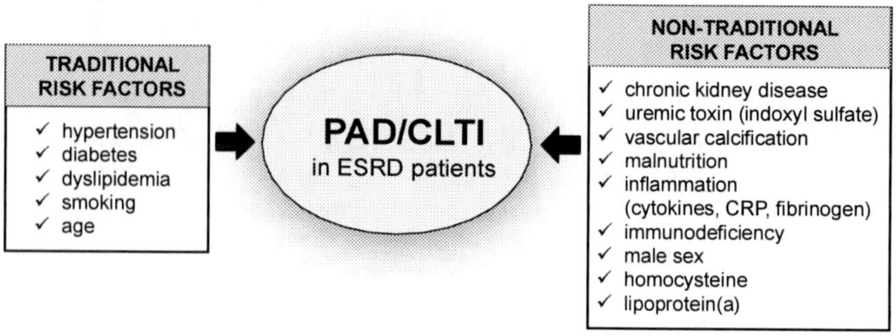

Figure 2. Risk factors for PAD/CLTI.
Abbreviations: PAD (peripheral artery disease); CLTI (critical limb-threatening ischemia); CRP (C-reactive protein);CKD (chronic kidney disease); ESRD (end-stage renal disease).

ABI is widely used for the screening test for PAD and is a useful measure for detecting PAD also in HD patients. However, it did not correlate with the severity among HD patients with PAD. In patients with noncalcified vessels, ABI often adequately indicates the severity of ischemia. However, ABI values might be influenced by vascular calcification and may lead to misunderstanding of PAD in HD patients. We evaluated the association between ABI and PAD in HD patients, and the best cut-off value of ABI for detecting PAD was at <1.06 in cases of HD patients (sensitivity of 80% and specificity of 98.0%) [24]. The levels of ABI did not significantly decrease along with the progression of PAD in HD patients (Table 1). Although ABI indicates the presence of PAD, ABI alone should not be used to assess the severity of the disease in patients with highly calcified vessels. The toe brachial index (TBI) was better correlated with the progression of PAD than ABI [24]. The TBI decreased along with the progression of PAD (Table 1). In consideration of the decrease of TBI with unparalleled ABI along with the progression of PAD, below-ankle arterial occlusion or stenosis was suggested to be important for the progression of PAD in HD patients and might be targeted for treatment. The skin perfusion pressure (SPP) is another screening method for detecting PAD and a predictor of the possibility of wound healing [37]. SPP measures the skin perfusion just beneath the skin and is not influenced by vascular calcification. In HD patients, the sensitivity and specificity of ABI < 0.9 for detecting PAD were 29.9% and 100%, whereas those in SPP < 50 mmHg were 84.9% and 76.6%, respectively [31]. For screening PAD in HD patients, SPP has a better sensitivity than ABI.

Table 1. Prevalence of polyvascular disease and ABI/TBI in HD patients (Ref.23).

	PAD(-)	PAD(+)		
		Fontaine classification		
	(n = 51)	I (n = 27)	II (n = 8)	IV (n = 11)
IHD (%)	9.8	55.6*	50.0*	54.5*
stroke (%)	3.9	22.2*	37.5*	36.3*
ABI	1.21 ± 0.09	0.92 ± 0.22*	0.82 ± 0.27	0.82 ± 0.26
TBI	0.78 ± 0.22	0.50 ± 0.24*	0.49 ± 0.21	0.16 ± 0.13**, ***

Abbreviations: PAD (peripheral artery disease); IHD (ischemic heart disease); ABI (ankle brachial index); TBI (toe brachial index).

* P < 0.01 vs. PAD(-), ** P < 0.01 vs. Fontaine I, *** p < 0.01 vs. Fontaine II.

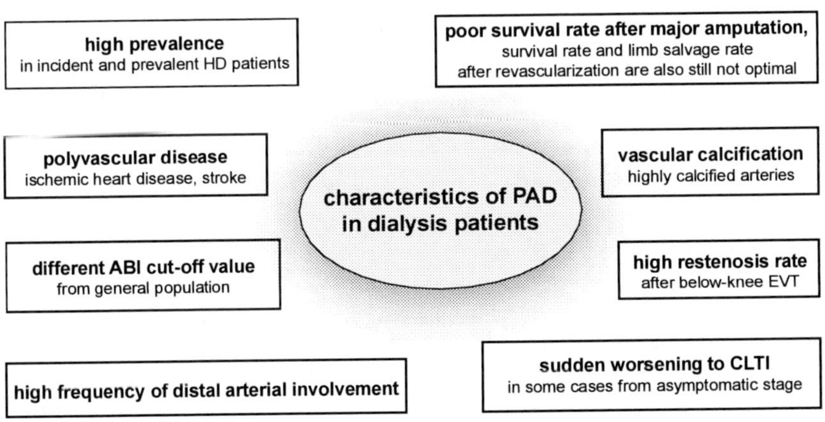

Figure 3. Characteristic features of PAD in dialysis patients.
Abbreviations: ABI, ankle brachial index;PAD, peripheral artery disease; EVT, endovascular therapy.

PAD at the initiation of HD is an independent risk factor for death [38]. The survival rate and limb salvage rate of HD patients with ischemic foot ulcers are 65.2% and 68.9% in 1 year and 23.4% and 53.8% in 5 years, respectively [39]. The survival rate after major amputation due to limb ischemia is 51.9% in 1 year and 14.4% in 5 years [40]. HD was observed to be an independent risk factor for death within 3 years after infrainguinal endovascular therapy (Hazard ration 2.91) [41]. Approximately one third of HD patients who underwent below-knee arterial revascularization died within 1 year [42]. The 1-year amputation-free survival rate after below-knee revascularization is 65.7% in EVT [43] and 60% in distal bypass surgery, respectively [44]. Even though EVT was successfully performed, the restenosis rate is significantly high in HD patients in cases of below-knee intervention (73% at 3 months and 82% at 12 months) [45]. In any case, the survival rate, limb salvage rate, amputation-free survival rate in HD patients who undergo revascularization therapy are significantly poor compared with those in non-dialysis patients [46]. The clinical characteristics of PAD in HD patients is summarized in Figure 3.

Conclusion

With the aging of the global population and increase of high-risk patients with diabetes and/or advanced stages of CKD (dialysis population), it seems likely that PAD will be increasingly more common in the future. PAD is strongly associated with mortality and worsens the quality of life. Although re-vascularization therapy is essential for patients with CLTI, the efficacy of revascularization therapy is regretfully still not optimal.

References

[1] Fowkes F. G. R. Rudan D. Rudan I. Aboyans V. Denenberg J. O. Mcdermott M. M. Norman P. E. Sampson U. K. A. Williams L. J. Mensah G. A. Criqui M. H. (2013). Comparison of global estimates of prevalence and risk factors for peripheral artery disease in 2000 and 2010: a systematic review and analysis. *Lancet* 382, 1329-40.

[2] Belch J. J. F. Topol E. J. Agnelli G. Bertrand M. Califf R. M. Clement D. L. Creager M. A. Easton J. D. Gavin 3 J. R. Greenland P. Hankey G. Hanrath P. Hirsh A. T. Meyer J. Smith S. C. Sullivan F. Weber M. A. (2003). Critical issues in peripheral arterial disease detection and management. *Arch Int Med* 163, 884-92.

[3] Asahara T. Murohara T. Sullivan A. Silver M. van der Zee R. Li T. Witzenbichler B. Schatterman G. Isner J. M. (1997). Isolation of putative progenitor endothelial cells for angiogenesis *Science* 275, 964-967.

[4] Suzuki H. Ohtake T. Tsukiyama T. Morota M. ishioka K. Moriya H. Mochida Y. Hidaka S. Sato T. Asahara T. Kobayashi S. (2021). Acute kidney injury successfully treated with autologous granulocyte colony-stimulating factor-mobilized peripheral

blood CD34-positive cell transplantation: A first-in-human report. *Stem Cells Transl Med* 10, 1253-7.

[5] Lee M. S. Lee F. Y. Chen Y. L. Sung P. H. Chaing H. J. Chen K. H. Huang T. H. Chen Y. L. Chaing J. Y. Yin T. C. Chang H. W. Yip H. K. (2017). Investigated the safety of intra-renal arterial transfusion of autologous CD34+ cells and time course of creatinine levels, endothelial dysfunction biomarkers and micro-RNAs in chronic kidney disease patients-phase I clinical trial. *Oncotarget* 8, 17750-62.

[6] Yang C. C. Sung P. H. Cheng B. C. Li Y. C. Chen Y. L. Lee M. S. Yip H. K. (2020). Safety and efficacy of intrarenal arterial autologous CD34+ cell transfusion in patients with chronic kidney disease: A randomzied, open-label controlled phase 2 clinical trial. *Stem Cells Transl Med* 9, 827-838.

[7] Sharma M. Rao P. N. Sasikala M. Kuncharam M. R. Reddy C. Gokak V. Raju B. Singh J. R. Nag P. Reddy D. N. (2015). Autologous mobilized peripheral blood CD34(+) cell infusion in non-viral decompensated liver cirrhosis. *World J Gastroenterol* 21, 7264-71.

[8] Al-Zoubi A. Jafar E. Jamous M. Al-Twai F. Al-Bakheet S. Zalloum M. Khalufeh F. Radi S. A. El-Khateeb M. Al-Zoubi Z. (2014). Transplantation of purified autologous leukapheresis-derived CD34+ and CD133+ stem cells for patients with chronic spinal cord injuries: long-term evaluation of safety and efficacy. *Cell Transplant* 23 Suppl 1, S25-34.

[9] Song P. Rudan D. Zhu Y. Fowkes F. J. I. Rahimi K. Fowkes G. R. Rudan I. (2019). Global, regional, and national prevalence and risk factors for peripheral artery disease in 2015: an updated systematic review and analysis. *Lancet Glob Health* 2019: 7: e1020-30.

[10] O'Hare A. M. Glidden D. V. Fox C. S. Hsu Chi-yuan, (2004). High prevalence of peripheral arterial disease in persons with renal insufficiency. Results from the national health and nutrition examination survey 1999-2000. *Circulation* 109, 320-3.

[11] Nehler M. R. Duval S. Diao L. Annex B. H. Hiatt W. R. Rogers K. Zakharyan A. Hirsch A. T. (2014). Epidemiology of peripheral arterial disease and critical limb ischemia in an insured national population. *J Vasc Surg* 60, 686-95.

[12] Takahara M. Iida O. Kohsaka S. Soga Y. Fijiwara M. Shinke T. Amano T. Ikari Y. J-EVT and J-PCI investigators. (2019). Diabetes mellitus and other cardiovascular risk factors in lower-extremity peripheral artery disease versus coronary artery disease: an analysis of 1,121,359 cases from the nationwide databases. *Cardiovasc Diabetol* 18, 155.

[13] Hicks C. W. Yang C. Ndumele C. E. Folsom A. R. Heiss G. Black 3rd J. H. Selvin E. Matsushita K. (2018). Association of obesity with incident hospitalization related to peripheral artery disease and critical limb ischemia in the ARIC study. *J Am Heart Assoc* 7, e008644.

[14] Bhatt D. L. Steg P. G. Ohman E. M. Hirsch A. T. Ikeda Y. Mas J. L. Goto S. Liau C. S. Richard A. J. Rother J. Wilson P. W. F. for the REACH Registry Investigators, (2006). International prevalence, recognition, and treatment of cardiovascular risk factors in outpatients with atherothrombosis. *JAMA* 295, 180-9.

[15] Sartipy F. Sigvant B. Lundin F. Wahlberg E. (2018). Ten-year mortality in different peripheral arterial disease stages: A population based observational study on outcome. *Eur J Vasc Endovasc Surg* 55, 529-36.

[16] Norgan L. Hiatt W. R. Dormandy J. A. Nehler M. R. Harris K. A. Fowkes F. G. R. TASC 2 Working Group, (2007). Inter-society consensus for the management of peripheral arterial disease (TASC II). *J Vasc Surg* 45, Suppl S, S5-67.

[17] Adams D. J. Beard J. D. Cleveland T. Brandbury A. W. Forbes J. F. Fowkes F. G. R. Gillepsie I. Ruckley C. V. Raab G. Storkey H. BASIL trial participants. (2007). Bypass versus angioplasty in severe ischemia of the leg (BASIL): multicenter, randomizes controlled trial. *Lancet* 366, 1925-34.

[18] Abu Dabrh A. M. Steffen M. W. Undavalli C. Asi N. Wang Z. Elamin M. B. Conte M. S. Murad M. H. (2015). The natural history of untreated severe or critical limb ischemia. *J Vasc Surg* 62, 1642-51.

[19] O'Hare A. M. Vittinghoff E. Hsia J. Shripak M. G. (2004). Renal insufficiency and the risk of lower extremity peripheral arterial disease: Results from the heart and estrogen/progestin replacement stusy (HERS). *J Am Soc Nephrol* 15, 1046-51.

[20] Kobayashi S. (2016). Cardiovascular events in chronic kidney disease (CKD) - an importance of vascular calcification and microcirculatory impairment. *Renal Replacement Therapy* 2, 55.

[21] Ohtake T. Kobayashi S. (2017). Impact of vascular calcification on cardiovascular mortality in hemodialysis patients: clinical significance, mechanisms and possible strategies for treatment. *Renal Replacement Therapy* 3, 13.

[22] Lin T. Y. Chou H. H. Huang H. L. Hung S. C. (2020). Indoxyl sulfate and incident peripheral artery disease in hemodialysis patients. *Toxins* 12, 696.

[23] Ohtake T. Oka M. Ikee R. Mochida Y. Ishioka K. Moriya H. Hidaka S. Kobayashi S. (2011). Impact of lower limbs' arterial calcification on the prevalence and severity of PAD in patients on hemodialysis. *J Vasc Surg* 53, 676-83.

[24] Kobayashi S. Oka M. Maesato K. Ikee R. Mano T. Moriya H. Ohtake T. (2008). Coronary artery calcification, ADMA, and insulin resistance in CKD patients. *Clin J Am Soc Nephrol* 3, 1289-95.

[25] O'hare A. M. Hsu C. Y. Bacchetti P. Johansen K. L. (2002). Peripheral vascular disease risk factors among patients undergoing hemodialysis. *J Am Soc Nephrol* 13, 497-503.

[26] Sueta D. Hokimoto S. Sakamoto K. Akasaka T. Tabata N. Kaikita K. Honda O. Naruse M. Ogawa H. Multicenter Study of Hemodialysis Patients Undergoing Invasive Cardiovascular Procedures Study Investigators, (2017). Validation of the high mortality rate of malnutrition-inflammation-atherosclerosis syndrome: - community-based observational study. *Int J Cardiol* 230, 97-102.

[27] Kalantar-Zadeh K. Stenvinkel P. Pillion L. Kopple J. D. (2003). Inflammation and nutrition in renal insufficiency. *Adv Ren Replace Ther* 10, 155-169.

[28] Shiraki T. Iida O. Takahara M. Soga Y. Yamauchi Y. Hirano K. Kawasaki D. Fijihara M. Utsunomiya M. Tazaki J. Yamaoka T. Shintani Y. Suematsu N. Suzuki K. Miyashita Y. Tsuchiya T. Uematsu M. (2015). Predictors of delayed wound healing after endovascular therapy of isolated infrapopliteal lesions underlying

critical limb ischemia in patients with high prevalence of diabetes mellitus and hemodialysis. *Eur J Vasc Endovasc Surg* 49, 565-73.

[29] Tian S. L. Zhang K. Xu P. C. (2018). Increased prevalence of peripheral arterial disease in patients with obese sarcopenia undergoing hemodialysis. *Exp Ther Med* 15, 5148-52.

[30] Ishioka K. Ohtake T. Moriya H. Mochida Y. Oka M. Maesato K. Hidaka S. Kobayashi S. (2018). High prevalence of peripheral arterial disease (PAD) in incident hemodialysis patients: screening by ankle-brachial index (ABI) and skin perfusion pressure (SPP) measurement. *Renal replacement Therapy* 4, 27.

[31] Okamoto K. Oka M. Maesato K. Ikee R. Mano T. Moriya H. Ohtake T. Kobayashi S. (2006). Peripheral arterial occlusive disease is more prevalent in patients with hemodialysis: comparison with the findings of multidetector-row computed tomography. *Am J Kidney Dis* 48, 269-76.

[32] Ono K. Tsuchida A. Kawai H. Matsuo H. Wakamatsu R. Maezawa A. Yano S. Kawada T. Nojima Y. (2003). Ankle-brachial blood pressure index predicts all-cause and cardiovascular mortality in hemodialysis patients. *J Am Soc Nephrol* 14, 1591-8.

[33] Koch M. Trapp R. Kulas W. Grabensee B. (2004). Critical limb ischemia as a main cause of death in patients with end-stage renal disease: a single centre study. *Nephrol Dial Transplant* 19, 2547-52.

[34] Azuma N. Kikuchi S. Okuda H. Miyake K. Koya A. (2017). Recent progress of bypass surgery to the dialysis-dependent patients with critical limb ischemia. *Ann Vasc Dis* 10, 178-84.

[35] Iida O. Namakura M. Yamauchi Y. Kawasaki D. Yokoi Y. Yokoi H. Soga Y. Zen K. Hirano K. Suematsu N. Inoue N. Suzuki K. Shintani Y. Miyashita Y. Urasawa K. Kitano I. Yamaoka T. Murakami T. Uesugi M. Tsuchiya T. Shinke T. Oba Y. Ohura N. Hamasaki T. Nanto S. OLIVE investigators, (2013). Endovascular treatment for infrainguinal vessels in patients with critical limb ischemia: OLIVE registry, a prospective, multicenter study in Japan with 12-month follow-up. *Circ Cardiovasc Interv* 6, 68-76.

[36] Takahara M. Iida O. Soga Y. Kodama A. Azuma N. (2015). Absence of preceding intermittent claudication and its associated clinical features in patients with critical limb ischemia. *J Atheroscler Thromb* 22, 718-25.

[37] Castroneuvo J. J. Adera H. M. Smiell J. M. Price R. M. (1997). Skin perfusion pressure measurement is valuable in the diagnosis of critical limb ischemia. *J Vasc Surg* 26, 629-37.

[38] Morooka H. Tanaka A. Inaguma D. Maruyama S. (2020). Peripheral artery disease at the time of dialysis initiation and mortality: a prospective observational multi-center study. *BMJ Open* 10, e042315.

[39] Orimoto Y. Ohta T. Ishibashi H. Sugimoto I. Iwata H. Yamada T. Tadakoshi M. Hida M. (2013). The prognosis of patients on hemodiaysis with foot lesions. *J Vasc Surg* 58, 1291-9.

[40] Aulivola B. Hile C. N. Hamdan A. D. Sheahan M. G. Veraldi J. R. Skillman J. J. Campbell D. R. Scovell S. D. LoGerfo F. W. Pomposelli Jr. F. B. (2004). Major lower extremity amputation: outcome of a modern series. *Arch Surg* 139, 395-9.

[41] Iida O. Namakura M. Yamauchi Y. Fukunaga M. Yokoi Y. Yokoi H. Soga Y. Zen K. Suematsu N. Inoue N. Suzuki K. Hirano K. Shintani Y. Miyashita Y. Urasawa K. Kitano I. Tsuchiya T. Kawamoto K. Yamaoka T. Uesugi M. Shinke T. Oba Y. Ohura N. Uematsu M. Takahara M. Hamasaki T. Nanto S. OLIVE Investigators, (2015). 3-year outcomes of the OLIVE registry, a prospective multicenter study of patients with critical limb ischemia: A prospective, multicenter, three-year follow-ups study on endovascular treatment for infra-inguinal vessel in patients with critical limb ischemia. *JACC Cardiovasc Interv* 8, 1493-1502.

[42] Suematsu N. Iida O. Takahara M. Yamauchi Y. Soga Y. Nakano M. Hirano K. Kawasaki D. Yamaoka T. Suzuki K. Shintani Y. Miyashita Y. Tazaki J. Meno H. Inou T. (2015). Prognostic factors in hemodialysis patients undergoing endovascular treatment for critical limb ischemia due to isolated below-the-knee disease. *J Atheroscler Thromb* 22, 404-14.

[43] Nakano M. Hirano K. Iida O. Yamauchi Y. Soga Y. Kawasaki D. Tazaki J. Suzuki K. Fujiwara M. Yamaoka T. (2015). Clinical efficacy of inftapopliteal endovascular procesures for hemodialysis patients with critical limb ischemia. *Ann Vasc Surg* 29, 1225-34.

[44] Kumada Y. Nogaki H. Ishii H. Aoyama T. Kamoi D. Takahashi H. Murohara T. (2015). Clinical outcome after infrapopliteal bypass surgery in chronic hemodialysis patients with critical limb ischemia. *J Vasc Surg* 61, 400-4.

[45] Iida O. Soga Y. Kawasaki D. Hirano K. Yamaoka T. Suzuki K. Miyashita Y. Yokoi H. Takahara M. Uematsu M. (2012). Angiographic restenosis and its clinical impact after infrapopliteal angioplasty. *Eur J Cardiovasc Surg* 44, 425-31.

[46] Dawson D. B. Telles-Garcia N. A. Atkins J. L. Abreo A. P. Virk C. S. Dominic P. S. (2021). End-stage renal disease patients undergoing angioplasty and bypass for critical limb ischemia have worse outcomes compared to non-ESRD patients: systematic review and meta-analysis. *Cather Cardiovasc Interv* 98, 297-307.

Section III: EPC in Metabolic Diseases

Chapter 4

Endothelial Progenitors in Metabolic Diseases

Mattia Albiero* **and Gian Paolo Fadini**
Department of Medicine, University of Padova, Padova, Italy
Veneto Institute of Molecular Medicine,
Experimental Diabetology Lab, Padova, Italy

Abstract

Endothelial progenitors have been described as circulating cells endowed with pro-angiogenic features that are believed to play an important role in cardiovascular homeostasis. Metabolic diseases are characterized by a two- to four-fold increased risk of cardiovascular disease due to the onset of microvascular and macrovascular dysfunctions. Preventing the onset of endothelial dysfunction in patients with metabolic diseases can be achieved through pharmacological therapies, aimed to improve the metabolic control while controlling the failure of endothelial function. The discovery of endothelial progenitors allowed to overturn this, speculating that endothelial damage might be the result of an exhaustion or a dysfunction of the pool of circulating progenitors, resulting in an impaired regenerative capacity. However, endothelial progenitors are circulating cells; therefore, their reduction by 30–50% in individuals with metabolic diseases was mechanistically proposed to be a defect of their release or, possibly, exhaustion of the bone marrow reservoir. This revolutionary concept, which placed the bone marrow at the central stage in the cardiometabolic field, will be examined thoroughly. The last part of the chapter will look at the endothelial progenitors from the patient's perspective, discussing whether their count in the peripheral blood could

* Corresponding Author's Email: mattia.albiero@unipd.it

In: Endothelial Progenitor Cells in Health and Disease
Editors: Amankeldi A. Salybekov, Shuzo Kobayashi and Takayuki Asahara
ISBN: 978-1-68507-794-5

be used as a cardiovascular biomarker, which could improve risk stratification and ultimately guide patient treatment. We will also address the potential benefits of current pharmacotherapy in the management of metabolic diseases to restore the endothelial progenitor count and functions.

In the final paragraph, we will review the lessons learned from cell-based trials for therapeutic neovascularization, trying to highlight the challenges of using endothelial progenitor for cell therapy in the contest of metabolic diseases.

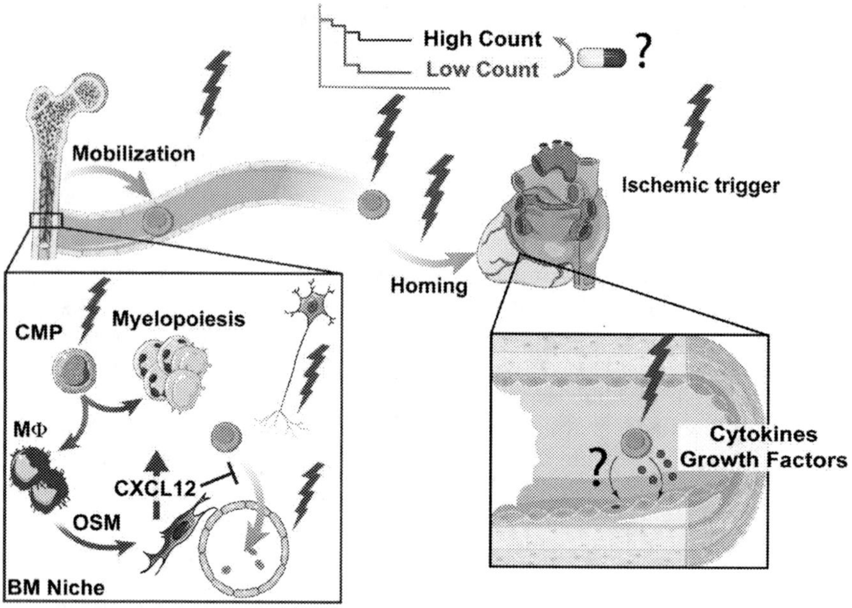

Graphical Abstract. Endothelial progenitors are circulating cells endowed with pro-angiogenic potential. A reduction by 30–50% in individuals with metabolic diseases is the result of a defect of their release from the bone marrow and, possibly, an exhaustion of their reservoir. Furthermore, impaired recruitment at site of neo-vascularization is also a feature of metabolic diseases. From the patient's perspective, the outcomes of the current pharmacotherapy in restoring endothelial progenitor count and functions are still a matter of investigation.

Keywords: diabetes, bone marrow, regeneration, risk factor

Introduction

In the wake of a decade where adult stem cell research was growing at an incredible pace, the identification of putative endothelial progenitors in 1997 as a subset of circulating $CD34^+$ cells, represented a turning point for the field [1].

Endothelial progenitors were initially described as "exceedingly rare" adult remnants of the elusive embryonic progenitors, known as hemangioblasts [2]; however, as the field moved forward, this hypothesis became less solid [3, 4]. During embryonic development, a small population of endothelial cells, termed hemogenic endothelial cell, localized within the murine yolk sac and aorta - gonad - mesonephros, transiently acquires the hematopoietic potency to initiate definitive hematopoiesis [5]. Evidence that the hemangioblast persists in the adult, or that mature endothelial cells retain hematopoietic activity are still debated. However, recent studies showed that, even in the embryo, after the differentiation from the hemogenic endothelium, hematopoietic progenitor cells cannot differentiate back into endothelial cells [6].

Over the last 25 years, the scientific community struggled to reach a shared definition of endothelial progenitors and a clear assessment of their true regenerative potential [7]. The most rigorous definition of endothelial progenitors should describe their phenotype and their biological functions. The critical re-evaluation of the culture protocols allowed to establish that endothelial progenitors cultured from the peripheral blood mononuclear cells (PBMCs) can differentiate into two different subsets of cells. Myeloid angiogenic cells, also known as circulating angiogenic cells (CACs), are cells of hematopoietic lineage endowed with a strong paracrine activity that, however, do not differentiate into true endothelial cells. Endothelial colony forming cells (ECFCs) are a subset of endothelial cells with an intrinsic angiogenic capacity, capable of vascular repair as well as *de novo* blood vessel formation [7].

To assess and quantify the endothelial progenitors in the clinical setting, flow cytometry has been the gold standard since the beginning. Following the landmark paper of Asahara et al. [1], cells expressing CD34 and vascular endothelial growth factor receptor 2 (VEGFR-2 also known as KDR in humans) were deemed as endothelial progenitors. Since CD34 can be expressed also by endothelial cells, some authors suggested that using the stem cell marker CD133 will cause the enrichment for more immature progenitors [8], although a subsequent work showed that $CD34^+KDR^+CD133^+$ cells are enriched in hematopoietic progenitors devoid of definite endothelial commitment [3].

The concept that circulating progenitor cells could contribute to endothelial homeostasis represented a turning point for vascular biology: it provided the foundation to generate a new pathophysiological hypothesis for cardiovascular diseases (CVD), to establish endothelial progenitors as a new biomarker for cardiovascular health, and to exploit them as a possible source for cell therapy [9].

Metabolic diseases, by definition, represent the pathological skewing from homeostasis of metabolic processes, either at the cellular or systemic level. Metabolic diseases can be due to inherited genetic mutations usually resulting in the lack of a specific enzyme, which causes a pathological accumulation of metabolites and byproducts that are toxic or interfere with the normal biological functions. The focus of this chapter, though, will be on acquired metabolic diseases, also known as metabolic disorders, such as diabetes, obesity, or dyslipidemia, which can have a strong genetic background, but are largely contributed to by overfeeding, aging, or environmental factors.

Notably, Fabry disease, an X-chromosomal recessive deficiency of the lysosomal hydrolase α-galactosidase A, characterized by increased cardiovascular risk and small vessel disease of the kidney, was associated with an impaired function of circulating angiogenic cells, which could be reverted by enzyme replacement therapy [10].

Acquired metabolic diseases are characterized by a two- to four-fold increased risk of CVD due to the onset of microvascular and macrovascular dysfunction. Microvascular dysfunction is mainly triggered by hyperglycemia-driven damages [11] while macrovascular dysfunction is initiated by endothelial dysfunction, resulting in accelerated atherosclerosis. In diabetic patients, approximately 60% of the excess mortality is due to cardiovascular complications; however, the risk of death associated with other diseases is also higher compared to subjects without diabetes [12]. The SARS-CoV-2 pandemic has once more identified diabetes as a high-risk condition due to the underlying low-grade inflammation and multi-organ damage [13]. The global prevalence of diabetes and obesity, sometimes described as the "diabesity pandemic," is a serious concern for all healthcare systems, since alarming reports project a rise in its prevalence and incidence in the subsequent years [14]. Indeed, while most therapies are effective in lowering the blood glucose, they are less able to prevent excess death among diabetic patients, which are plagued by the token of chronic complications. As of yet, chronic diabetic complications like retinopathy, neuropathy, and delayed wound healing do not have a definite or dedicated treatment.

In the following paragraphs, we will describe the alterations of endothelial progenitors in metabolic diseases and the central role played by the bone marrow in this process. Next, we will discuss the role of endothelial progenitors as biomarkers for cardiovascular health and, finally, the challenges of using endothelial progenitors, and pro-angiogenic progenitors in general, as a source for cell therapy in metabolic diseases.

Endothelial Progenitor Cell Alteration in Metabolic Diseases

At a physiological level, the endothelium promotes vasodilation, fibrinolysis, and anti-aggregation, thus preventing the onset of CVD [15]. It is generally accepted that in diabetes a plethora of molecular and cellular events trigger endothelial dysfunction, promoting aggregation, reducing NO release, and ultimately increasing the cardiovascular risk [16]. While hyperglycemia-derived reactive oxygen species (ROS) have been described as the major driver for microvascular dysfunction [17], the mechanisms underlying endothelial dysfunction in macrovascular complications, such as atherosclerosis, encompass a more complex scenario, which includes hyperglycemia, a pro-inflammatory environment, and insulin resistance.

Preventing the onset of endothelial dysfunction in patients with metabolic diseases can be achieved through pharmacological therapies that aim to improve metabolic control while reducing the failing of endothelial function. Endothelial progenitors allowed to overturn this prospective, speculating that endothelial damage might be the result of an exhaustion or a dysfunction of the pool of circulating progenitors, resulting in an impaired regenerative capacity [18]. Indeed, the yield of endothelial progenitors cultured from PBMCs of type 1 and type 2 diabetic patients was lower compared to healthy controls, and diabetic endothelial progenitors performed significantly worse in angiogenic assays *in vitro* [19, 20]. However, it was conceptually and clinically important to confirm these findings *in vivo*, using flow cytometry. Our group consistently showed that $CD34^+KDR^+$ cells are reduced in the peripheral blood of diabetic patients; additionally, this reduction is worsened in patients with peripheral vascular complications [21-23]. In obese patients, even without diabetes, the number of $CD34^+KDR^+$ cells were reduced and their angiogenic potency was impaired, but after weight loss, the $CD34^+KDR^+$ counts significantly improved [24-26].

The investigation for endothelial progenitor dysfunction in diabetes, initially followed the same conceptual framework used to study endothelial dysfunction [27]. Endothelial progenitors, however, are circulating cells that are supposedly released from the bone marrow to home at sites where physiological angiogenesis or vascular regeneration might occur [28]. This concept introduced the possibility that the dysfunction of the endothelial progenitor in metabolic diseases was due, also, to an impaired recruitment at the sites of vascular injury associated with an impaired release from the bone marrow.

Intrinsic Defect of Endothelial Progenitors in Metabolic Diseases

Hyperglycemia was consistently reported as one of most common noxae that impaired the yield of endothelial progenitor *in vitro* [19] and optimized glycemic control was followed by an improved $CD34^+KDR^+$ cells count in patients [29].

During the natural history of type 2 diabetes, carbohydrate metabolism progressively worsened from normal glucose tolerance, to impaired fasting glucose, and to impaired glucose tolerance, eventually leading to the diagnosis of type 2 diabetes. Notably, the decline of $CD34^+$ and $CD34^+KDR^+$ cells begin to occur very early in patients with impaired glucose intolerance, reaching a nadir at the diagnosis of type 2 diabetes [30]. As diabetes ensues, the decline in the progenitor cell count somehow stabilizes, possibly as a result of lifestyle changes imposed after a new diagnosis of diabetes, or due to antihyperglycemic drugs. After a disease duration of at least 20 years, there was a further reduction of circulating $CD34^+$ cells. Mechanistically, hyperglycemia was associated with increased generation of reactive oxygen species (ROS) through p66Shc [31], an adaptor protein which can propagate oxidative stress by mitochondrial uncoupling [32], although *in vitro* the main effect of high glucose was associated to an impaired bioavailability of nitric oxide (NO) rather than an excess of ROS [33]. However, in mice lacking p66Shc, endothelial cells were protected from hyperglycemic damage because of reduced oxidative stress [34] and because of the suppression of detrimental hyperglycemic memory [35]. Notably, in human PBMC of diabetic patients, the mRNA for p66Shc is upregulated [36], suggesting that the role of p66Shc might be relevant also in patients. *In vitro*, high glucose impaired the angiogenic features of endothelial progenitors, increased apoptosis, decreased

MMP-9 activity, and NO release [33]. Nevertheless, in patients with marked hyperglycemia, the apoptotic $CD34^+$ cells count was comparable to healthy subjects, but in patients with type 2 diabetes, a negative correlation was observed between the peripheral blood $CD34^+$ cells count and $CD34^+$ cell apoptosis [30]. Relevant to the pro-inflammatory environment associated with type 2 diabetes, TNF-α increased in a time- and dose-dependent fashion p38-MAPK signaling *in vitro*, reducing the endothelial progenitor number [37]. The endothelial progenitors from patients with coronary artery disease (CAD) had higher levels of p38-phosphorylation compared with healthy subjects.

Table 1. Summary of clinical studies reporting endothelial progenitor alterations in metabolic diseases

Diabetes		
Reference	Endothelial progenitor phenotype and alterations	Clinical correlations
[145]	Reduced $CD34^+$ and $CD34^+KDR^+$ cells in newly diagnosed diabetes. Reduced $CD34^+$ cells in prediabetes	Negative correlations with fasting and post-challenge glucose
[90]	Components of the Metabolic Syndrome were associated by reduction of $CD34^+$ cells and acted synergistically in decreasing $CD34^+$ cell count	Negative correlation between $CD34^+$ cells and CV risk
[30]	Early decline of $CD34^+$ cells after the onset of type 2 diabetes, and progressive reduction during the natural history of the disease	Negative correlation between PB $CD34^+$ cell count and apoptotic $CD34^+$ cells. Direct correlation between PB and BM and $CD34^+$ cell counts
[19]	Reduced yield of cultured $acLDL^+$-$lectin^+$-$CD31^+$ cells from type 1 diabetic patients	Negative correlation with Hb1Ac
[146]	Reduction of multiple phenotype of endothelial progenitors in type 2 diabetes markers	Multiple negative correlation with different diabetic complications and disease severity
[20]	Reduced yield and function of cultured $acLDL^+$-$lectin^+$ cells from type 2 diabetic patients	Negative correlation with Hb1Ac and diabetes duration
Obesity		
[26]	Reduced $CD34^+KDR^+$, $CD34^+CD133^+$, and $CD34^+$c-kit^+ cells in obese versus overweight subjects	Negative correlation between endothelial progenitors and BMI
[24]	Reduction of $CD34^+KDR^+$, $CD34^+CD133^+KDR^+$cells in obese patients	Negative correlation with BMI
	Reduced pro-angiogenic functions of $acLDL^+$-$lectin^+$ cultured endothelial progenitors in obese patients	No clinical correlation reported. The disfunction was reversible by inhibition of p38 MAPK

Table 1. (Continued)

Hypercholesterolemia		
Reference	Endothelial progenitor phenotype and alterations	Clinical correlations
[49]	Reduced $CD34^+CD133^+$ cells and impaired migration of cultured endothelial progenitors in patients with high LDL cholesterol	Inverse correlation between endothelial progenitors and LDL and direct correlation with HDL
[147]	Reduced $CD34^+KDR^+$ cells in hypercholesterolemic patients compared to normocholesterolemic subjects. Impaired	Inverse correlation with LDL cholesterol and aortic pulse wave velocity

Abbreviations. PB: peripheral blood. BM: bone marrow. BMI: body mass index.

Treatment with SB203580, an inhibitor of p38 mitogen-activated protein kinase (MAPK), resulted in an increased number of EPCs, *in vivo* and *in vitro*, and a reduction of cells expressing monocytic markers *in vitro* [38]. Hyperglycemia can skew the differentiation of endothelial progenitors *in vitro* toward macrophages and dendritic cells [39], and *in vivo* can rewire the bone marrow toward the generation of $CD11b^+CD45^{hi}CCR2^+Ly6C^{hi}$ inflammatory monocytes at the expenses of endothelial progenitors [40].

Lipotoxicity, often triggered by chronically elevated free fatty acid (FFA) levels, and hypercholesterolemia underlie the association between insulin resistance (and T2D), endothelial dysfunction, and increased CV risk [41]. Stearic acid, even at physiological concentrations, induced a pro-inflammatory response of pro-angiogenic cells *in vitro* along with increased apoptosis [42]. Similarly, hypercholesterolemic patients have a reduced number of circulating endothelial progenitors compared to normolipidemic ones [43]. Oxidized low-density lipoproteins induced endothelial progenitor senescence, decreased survival, and pro-angiogenic functions *in vitro*, through the activation of p38 MAPK [44-46]. In patients, the circulating $CD34^+KDR^+$ cells were negatively correlated with the LDL-cholesterol levels [47], although HDL-cholesterol appeared to be a strong determinant of the EPC number and function [48, 49]. Collectively, association studies and *in vitro* experiments showed that the intrinsic dysfunction of endothelial progenitors in metabolic diseases was driven by the same mechanism as that described for endothelial dysfunction (Table 1) [50]. However, endothelial cells are resident cells, while endothelial progenitors are by definition circulating cells that can be released from a reservoir compartment, such as the bone marrow. They then migrate, circulate into the bloodstream, and eventually home to the sites of vascular injury or inflammation [51]. This substantial difference allows the building of new hypotheses to explain the dysfunction of endothelial progenitors but, at the same time, obliges researchers to use more robust *in vivo* models to provide mechanistic data. This has opened a new field of studies, which are still very relevant today and will be discussed in the next paragraph.

Endothelial Progenitor Dysfunction as a Pathology of the Bone Marrow

Hematopoietic stem/progenitor cells (HSPCs) normally circulate in the peripheral blood (PB), accounting for about 0.05% of white blood cells (~3 cells/μl of blood). Circulating HSPCs are now known to be finely regulated by neuro-hormonal signals; however, the exact functions of HSPCs in PB remain elusive. As a subtype of HSPCs, endothelial progenitors should be subjected to a similar homeostatic regulation. Since the level of endothelial progenitors has been proposed to be indicative of a patient's endogenous vascular repair potential [52], the reduction of their level by 30–50% in individuals with diabetes, was mechanistically proposed to be a defect of their release or, possibly, and exhaustion of the bone marrow reservoir.

This hypothesis, despite being rather intuitive to explain the reduction in the peripheral circulation, was not initially fostered. In 2006, our group showed for the first time, in rats, that hind-limb ischemia, which represented a strong trigger for the release of endothelial progenitors, was completely ineffective in diabetic animals [53]. Ischemia triggers the activation of the HIF-1α pathway, which boosts the release of chemokine and growth factors, such as CXCL12, VEGF, and NO, which are essential for the mobilization of endothelial progenitors from the bone marrow [54]. In diabetes, ROS-induced modification of HIF1-α by the glyoxalase 1 (GLO1) substrate methylglyoxal, blocked the activation of this pathway upon ischemia, impaired the release of CXCL12 and VEGF, ultimately blunting the release of endothelial and hematopoietic progenitors [53, 55].

NO is a potent vasoactive molecule, which can induce vasodilation; however, it is also involved in compensatory angiogenesis following ischemia [56]. The mobilization of hematopoietic and endothelial progenitors requires the production of NO from endothelial and stroma cells of the bone marrow [57], and the reduced bioavailability of NO in diabetes has been linked to impaired endothelial progenitor mobilization and poor post-ischemic recovery [58]. Indeed, intracellular glucose flux causes mitochondrial overproduction of ROS, uncoupling endothelial nitric oxide synthase (eNOS) [16]. Furthermore, the reaction of ROS with NO leads to the production of peroxynitrite (ONOO-), which penetrates across the membranes and produces substrate nitration [34]. Therefore, a strategy to overcome the reduction of NO and restore the mobilization of endothelial progenitors might represent a valuable therapy.

These results showed that a defect signaling in the peripheral tissue is present in diabetes, resulting in a dampened release of endothelial progenitors. In the absence of an acute event, such as peripheral ischemia or myocardial infarction, the reduction in circulating progenitors reported in obese and diabetic patients cannot be explained by a defective trigger. On the contrary, if patients with metabolic disorders experience a failing cardiovascular system, a steady increase of endothelial progenitors should be expected. Therefore, investigations were put forward by different groups to address if a defect in the bone marrow was present and might explain the reduced level of endothelial progenitors. Indeed, by analyzing the bone marrow of type 2 diabetic rats, Busik et al. showed that the impaired release of endothelial progenitors from the diabetic bone marrow was caused by bone marrow neuropathy and that these changes precede the development of diabetic retinopathy [59]. In parallel, other structural alterations were reported in the bone marrow of type 1 diabetic animals, such as the exhaustion of stromal cells and the depletion of endothelial cells, leading to a form of microangiopathy [60, 61]. Importantly, endothelial and stromal cells are two paramount components of the hematopoietic stem cell niche [62].

We have shown that in the bone marrow of type 1 and type 2 diabetic mice, a neuropathic phenotype is associated with an impaired release of endothelial progenitor after ischemia [63]. Notably, diabetic p66Shc$^{-/-}$ mice were protected from bone marrow denervation and showed a rescued mobilization after ischemia. However, at the same time, p66Shc is required to trigger the mobilization cascade in the peripheral tissue [64]. The group of the late Paul Frenette [65] elegantly showed that the sympathetic nervous system of the bone marrow regulates the mobilization of HSPCs following granulocyte colony-stimulating factor (G-CSF), which is routinely used in patients to mobilize HSPCs in the peripheral blood, which will be collected by apheresis and transplanted for bone marrow reconstitution [66]. Therefore, we queried whether G-CSF - induced mobilization was defective in diabetes, due to this severe neuropathic phenotype. Indeed, we and others could show that G-CSF was completely ineffective in mobilizing HSPCs and endothelial progenitors in streptozotocin-induced diabetic mice [63, 67]. This defect in stem cell mobilization was termed as diabetic stem cell mobilopathy [68] and allowed us to envisage the bone marrow as a possible novel target of diabetic complications [69]. Similarly to what was seen in animal models, structural alterations were reported in human bone marrow biopsies [70]. Furthermore, a retrospective analysis of autologous stem cell transplantation procedures showed that diabetes was strongly associated with a poor-mobilizer phenotype [67]. All the data suggested that it was worth to test the daring hypothesis that diabetic stem cell mobilopathy was present also in humans. In a small but robust prospective clinical trial, we were the first to confirm that in diabetic patients a single injection of low-dose (5 μg/kg) human G-CSF was completely ineffective in mobilizing HSPCs and pro-angiogenic cells [71].

Among other pathways, mobilization is regulated by the CXCL12-CXCR4 axis. High levels of CXCL12 in the bone marrow retains HSPCs in the bone marrow niches, whereas inverting such gradients allows the egress of HSPCs and endothelial progenitors [72]. The gradient of CXCL12 is maintained also by the activity of dipeptidyl peptidase-4 (DPP-4), which by cleaving the amino terminal KP dipeptide from CXCL12 reduces its bioavailability [73]. At baseline, the DPP4 activity is higher in the peripheral blood compared to the bone marrow of diabetic compared to non-diabetic rats [51]. In response to G-CSF, DPP-4 activity in the bone marrow increased in non-diabetic but not in diabetic animals, allowing the switching of gradient of CXCL12, thus promoting mobilization [51].

Notably, diabetic patients, like diabetic mice, can mobilize HSPCs and endothelial progenitors upon stimulation with plerixafor (AMD3100), which is an antagonist of the CXCR4 receptor, thereby acting directly on HSPCs and endothelial progenitor cells [63, 74]. This last piece of evidence suggests that endothelial progenitors and HSPCs might be intrinsically responsive to mobilization, and that a major target in diabetes and metabolic diseases is indeed the bone marrow microenvironment.

Bone marrow macrophages are an important component of the hematopoietic stem cell niche, as they signal the stromal cells to retain HSPCs within the bone marrow [75]. Type 1 diabetic mice had increased $CD169^+$ bone marrow macrophages, which counteract G-CSF-induced mobilization of HSPCs [76]. By the secretion of Oncostatin M (OSM), macrophages trigger the expression of CXCL12 by bone marrow stromal cells, thus retaining HSPCs, and possibly endothelial progenitors, within the bone marrow. The expansion of bone marrow macrophages is possibly linked to the activation of myelopoiesis induced by hyperglycemia, which induces proliferation and expansion of bone marrow myeloid progenitors, prompting the release of monocytes into the circulation and fueling the onset of atherosclerosis [77]. Notably, we found that myelopoiesis is mechanistically linked to impaired mobilization, through an OSM-p66Shc pathway, driven by hyperglycemia [78]. It is important to understand, and possibly address, the mechanism of bone marrow dysfunction, since myelopoiesis is present also in models of type 2 diabetes, albeit less strikingly; however, mobilization is not affected both in $Lep^{Ob/Ob}$ mice and HFD-fed mice [79, 80].

The functional and structural alterations of the bone marrow are solid evidence in experimental metabolic diseases and could represent an additional mechanism to explain impaired release of endothelial progenitors (Figure 1). This hypothesis is supported in patients by the data gained from functional studies, such as mobilization assays, while the cellular and molecular mechanisms are still missing. It is important to note that a recent work challenged the hypothesis that endothelial progenitors originate from the bone marrow, by studying the phenotype of cultured endothelial progenitors isolated from male patients who had undergone allogeneic bone marrow transplant from female donors [81]. The authors showed that the early outgrowth fraction, which is usually enriched in cells endowed with strong pro-angiogenic activity, originated from the transplanted bone marrow, while $CD31^+$ cells in the late outgrowth fraction are likely derived from the recipient vasculature.

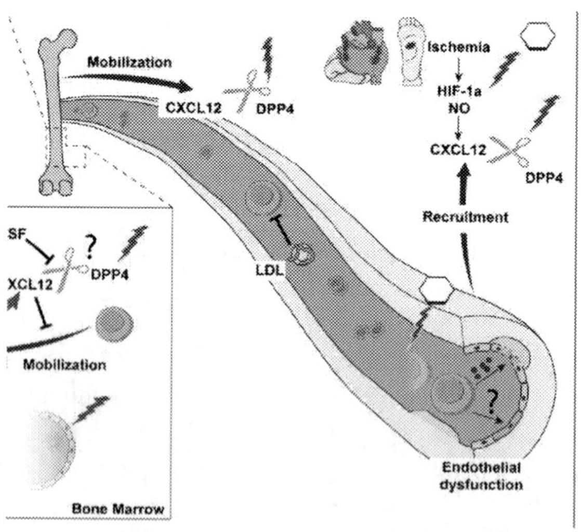

Figure 1. Mechanism of endothelial progenitor dysfunction in diabetes and metabolic diseases. The cartoon depicts how metabolic diseases in general (red lighting) or hyperglycemia (hexagon associated with red lightning) can impact endothelial progenitors at different layers, from deranging the bone marrow niche to deregulating their mobilization and recruitment at sites of vascular damage.

Endothelial Progenitors as a Cardiovascular Biomarker

Despite the controversies about the true regenerative potential of endothelial progenitors, the possibility to quantify them accurately and reproducibly in different cohorts of patients using flow cytometry could qualify them as a potential cardiovascular biomarker [82], which could improve the risk stratification [83] and ultimately guide patient treatment. The combination of antigens used to define endothelial progenitors should include at least 1 marker of stemness/immaturity (usually CD34 and/or CD133 in humans; CD34, c-kit, or Sca-1 in mice), plus at least 1 marker of endothelial commitment. The critical role of the CD34 as a marker is supported by the finding that the proangiogenic activity is lacking in selected CD34-negative cells [84]. After the original characterization, circulating endothelial progenitors have been defined as $CD34^+KDR^+$ by several investigators, as it was confirmed that this phenotype identifies cells capable of stimulating angiogenesis *in vivo* [85]. The number of circulating $CD34^+KDR^+$ cells is around 50–100/million WBC (0.005–0.01%), or 350–700 cells/mL. However, it has been criticized that this phenotype overlaps in part with that of hematopoietic stem/progenitor cells (which are $CD34^+$ and can express KDR) and with CECs (which are KDR^+ and may be $CD34^+$) [52]. To this end, the authors suggested that the co-expression of the stem cell antigen CD133, which is not expressed by mature endothelial cells, could increase the specificity for endothelial progenitor [52], although the frequency of $CD34^+CD133^+KDR^+$ cells in peripheral blood is about 20-fold lower, making quantification practically unreliable, unless millions of events are acquired (as is done for the screening of minimal residual disease). Therefore, complex antigenic phenotypes might provide information about the cells under investigation, but have lower reproducibility, thus limiting their use in clinical practice, resulting in an underperforming biomarker. Indeed, biomarkers that are statistically validated to be surrogates for a clinical endpoint could not be part of the pathophysiological process that results in that endpoint [82].

Another paramount feature of a biomarker is relevance, which refers to the ability of the biomarker to provide clinically pertinent information with predictive power. Patel et al. showed that $CD34^+$ mononuclear cells were associated with the risk of death in individuals at high cardiovascular risk and that both $CD34^+$ cells and $CD34^+/CD133^+$ cells are predictive of future adverse events [86]. Furthermore, Werner et al. followed-up patients with angiographically confirmed coronary artery disease (CAD), showing that $CD34^+KDR^+$ cells and $CD133^+$ cells were predictive of a first major cardiovascular event, independent of the potential confounders [87]. Upon pooling data from four longitudinal studies, our group showed that either $CD34^+$ cells or $CD34^+KDR^+$ cells help in identifying more patients at higher risk of future events over the short term [88].

In the contest of metabolic diseases, hypercholesterolemia, obesity, and diabetes have been associated with reduced circulating endothelial progenitors, even when using divergent methodologies, from a flow cytometry analysis to cell culture. Indeed, a linear correlation was also found between the severity of the risk factor and degree of endothelial progenitors count, which supports a causal link between the risk factors and endothelial progenitor reduction [52].

In patients with metabolic diseases and other conditions as well, multiple risk factors can occur at the same time; however, it is still not clear if a single risk factor or their combinations can negatively affect endothelial progenitors. However, few studies showed that endothelial progenitor cells progressively decrease as the number of risk factor increase [23, 47]. This is particularly notable in the contest of metabolic syndrome, which by definition is a constellation of risk factors for CVD and type 2 diabetes mellitus, which includes elevated waist circumference, elevated triglycerides, low high-density lipoprotein cholesterol, elevated blood pressure, and elevated fasting glucose. In patients, the clustering of risk factors, despite being of doubtful clinical usefulness, synergistically impaired the number of circulating $CD34^+$ cells [89, 90]. The remodeling of the bone marrow and the shortage of circulating endothelial progenitors could be a more general feature associated with accelerated aging and excess mortality described in diabetes. Indeed, low levels of HSPCs phenotypes (e.g. $CD34^+$ and $CD34^+CD133^+$) are independent determinants of all-cause mortality in different population of subjects, such as patients with metabolic syndrome, CVD or renal disease [52].

On the basis of the current literature, the CD34 and KDR antigenic combination represents a valuable cardiovascular biomarker and the best compromise in terms of sensitivity, specificity, and reliability to quantify endothelial progenitors in the clinical setting. It will be important to confirm the performance of endothelial progenitors as biomarkers in a lower-risk population as well. To this end, $CD34^+$ cells quantification is a routine analysis in most hematolology laboratories. Thus, it could be more easily applied in the clinical practice for CVD risk estimation, given its strong predictive power [90].

Diabetes Pharmacotherapy to Restore the Endothelial Progenitor Count and Function

A low endothelial progenitor count in the peripheral blood is a robust predictor for future cardiovascular events, even in the absence of metabolic diseases [91]. The clinical data support, but do not prove the idea that endothelial progenitors influence vascular complications and outcomes, since it is challenging to perform longitudinal clinical studies to assess the role of endothelial progenitors. However, several pre-clinical works supported the vascular tropism of human HSPCs [92] and showed that increase in the release of endothelial progenitors promoted vascular repairs in experimental diabetes [58]. Furthermore, in a cohort of patients with type 1 diabetes lasting for 50 years or longer, the level of circulating endothelial progenitors was higher in patients without CVD or nephropathy [93]. This association strengthened the hypothesis stating that preserving the endothelial progenitor number and function, or boosting the release from the bone marrow, could represent an additional endpoint in the treatment of patients with metabolic diseases.

As for other cardiovascular risk factors, lifestyle changes represent the first line of intervention that was shown to restore the endothelial progenitor count and function. A single bout and regular prolonged physical exercise can improve the circulating number and function of the endothelial progenitors, which was proposed to be mediated by the changes in circulating mediators, such as VEGF, G-CSF, and SDF-1α [94, 95]. Similarly, weight loss strategies in morbidly obese patients were associated with improved endothelial progenitor cell counts [95].

However, diabetic and metabolic patients are, in general, subjected to multiple pharmacological treatments aiming at each single risk factor to be brought to target [96]. Therefore, several therapies have been described to be associated with improving either the EPC number in patients or by enhancing their functional properties *in vitro* [97-99]. Statins, for instance, independently from their cholesterol lowering effects, can activate the protein kinase Akt in endothelial cells, which leads to the posttranscriptional activation of the eNOS via phosphorylation of Serine^{1177} [100, 101]. This mechanism was described to be relevant for inducing endothelial progenitor mobilization from the bone marrow [102, 103], to improve their yield and their angiogenic properties in culture [104-106] that improved reendothelializations in a model of vascular injury [107].

However, the most important group of drugs that have an impact on endothelial progenitors in the contest of metabolic diseases are glucose lowering drugs. Inverse correlations were demonstrated between glucose levels or HbA1c and circulating HSPCs or endothelial progenitors; thus, most studies consistently show that active glucose control can constrain the decline of stem/progenitor cells. Due to ethical concerns, most results were inferred from observational studies initially reporting the effect of glucose control achieved by means of insulin therapy, which showed that lowering of glucose levels can take several months to restore endothelial progenitors towards normal levels [108]. The majority of the studies concluded that regardless of the drug used, glucose control per se was effective in raising the levels of HSPCs and endothelial progenitors [109]. This evidence suggests that the underlying mechanisms rely on sustained hyperglycemic damages that, for instance, can skew the bone marrow microenvironment and HSPCs toward the generation of inflammatory cells, by the accumulation of advanced glycation end-products (AGEs) [77]. Among the glucose lowering drugs that can affect endothelial progenitors, the inhibitors of the dipeptidyl peptidase-4 (DPP-4i) are particularly notable [110]. They are widely used for the treatment of type 2 diabetes because they prevent the N-terminal cleavage and inactivation of incretin hormones, mainly GLP-1 (glucagon- like peptide-1) by DPP-4. Among the other physiological targets of this peptidase, the chemokine CXCL12/SDF-1α (stromal- derived factor-1α) represents a master determinant of HSPCs and endothelial progenitor traffic [54]. By preventing the enzymatic degradation of CXCL12, DPP-4i raises the concentrations of active CXCL12 in the periphery, leading to an increase in stem/progenitor cells [51]. Several molecules of the DPP-4i class have been shown to increase the levels of stem/progenitor cells in patients with diabetes, including sitagliptin compared to no treatment [111], voglibose [112], or glimepiride [112], vildagliptin compared to glibenclamide [113] and linagliptin [114].

This effect is rather rapid, since it occurs within just a few days and is correlated to the increased concentrations of active CXCL12 [111, 114]. A recent work, however, suggested that the cleavage of CXCL12 by CD26, which is the membrane bound form of DPP-4, did not appear to be a critical mechanism governing HSPCs trafficking in response to G-CSF [115]. Whether these findings are also relevant in steady-state conditions remain to be elucidated. Notably, saxagliptin had a direct protective effect on pro-angiogenic cells from T2D patients, since it reversed their dysfunction *in vitro* and improved inducible angiogenesis by circulating cells *in vivo* [116].

Glucose homeostasis is maintained through its renal resorption in the proximal tubule by the sodium glucose cotransporter-2 (SGLT-2). The inhibitors of SGLT-2 (SGLT2i) are a new class of drug aiming to improve glucose control by promoting urinary glucose excretion. SGLT-2 expression in the kidney is manifold compared to any other tissue [79], such that the effects of SGLT-2i are expected to be almost exclusively renal. In a small randomized controlled trial and in an observational study in T2D patients, neither the dapagliflozin or empagliflozin exerted a direct effect on HSPCs or endothelial progenitor levels; however, glucose control achieved by the means of SGLT2i, was able to raise the level of endothelial progenitors after several months of treatment [117]. On the other hand, another study suggested that empagliflozin could increase the levels of aldehyde dehydrogenase$^+$ progenitors, which the authors suggested were provided with vascular properties, although this discrepancy might be related to the methodological differences in the definition of endothelial progenitors [118]. Recently, we could demonstrate that in type 1 diabetic mice, the treatment with the SGLT2i dapagliflozin was able to reduce the frequency of CD169$^+$ macrophages in the bone marrow that are linked to impaired mobilization [76], thus reverting stem cell mobilopathy after stimulation with G-CSF [79]. In parallel, we were able to rescue the traffic of bone marrow (bone marrow)-derived cells to injured carotid arteries improving endothelial healing in mice. The relevance of these findings in humans, especially in patients with T2D is warranted. The role of CD169$^+$ macrophages in regulating endothelial progenitor and HSPCs trafficking, has proven to be relevant to explain one of the effects of PPAR-γ activation by thiazolidinediones (glitazones), a class of drugs used to improve the glycemic control and insulin resistance. Pioglitazone was found to be more effective in increasing the endothelial progenitor count, even in patients with well-controlled diabetes (109). We have provided evidence that PPAR-γ activation by pioglitazone could reprogram bone marrow macrophages toward an anti-inflammatory phenotype, reducing intra-marrow CXCL12 concentrations, thus favoring the mobilization of HSPCs in human and murine diabetes [119].

Despite the huge amount of data showing that the endothelial progenitor count can be achieved by improving glucose control or using glucose lowering drugs, there are several unresolved issues with important clinical counterparts. We still do not know how long the effects on endothelial progenitor are endured, and if a rather rapid mobilization triggered by a switch in the CXCL12 gradient translates into lasting increased levels of endothelial progenitors. Furthermore, the most striking gap is causal proof, beyond associative or predictive studies, that an increased level of endothelial progenitors or HSPCs improves the clinical outcomes. To test this hypothesis with a pharmacological approach, devoid of metabolic off-target effects, our group has recently performed a randomized double-blind placebo-controlled trial testing the mobilization of HSPCs with plerixafor (AMD3100) for the treatment of ischemic diabetic wounds, which was shown to be promising in a pre-clinical study [120]. Diabetic patients who received plerixafor on top of the standard of care, had a robust raise in the HSPC count, but displayed no improvement in wound healing compared to the placebo group [121], with a trend towards worse outcomes. While the small sample size could justify the results, it is possible that the transient mobilization triggered by plerixafor could not be sufficient to improve wound healing and, at the same time, it has been shown that ischemic tissues in diabetes had impaired expression of CXCL12, which is important to recruit HSPCs and endothelial progenitors [53, 55]. Indeed, wound healing in diabetic mice could be promoted by the on-site production and delivery of CXCL12 [122]. These findings, albeit negative, are revealing regarding the risks of translating pre-clinical findings to patients, especially in the context of metabolic diseases.

Despite robust evidence that several class of drugs, including glucose-lowering drugs, can increase the number or circulating HSPCs and endothelial progenitors, it has not been confirmed yet if this effect persists over time, because diabetic complications develop over several years; however, long-term studies are lacking. Therefore, the eventual benefits on chronic complications and on patient outcomes due to sustained elevation of endothelial progenitors or HSPCs count, should be demonstrated.

Challenges in Using Endothelial Progenitors for Cell Therapy in Patients with Metabolic Diseases

The idea to exploit endothelial progenitors as a source for autologous cell therapy to treat vascular diseases was translated into clinical trials remarkably soon, before the field reached a consensus about the true identity of endothelial progenitors and their regenerative potential. To be intellectually fair, it must be acknowledged that the enthusiasm and expectations for this approach might have stemmed, at least in part, from early studies showing remarkable effects of bone marrow cells infusion in pre-clinical models [123, 124], that could not be replicated independently by others [125]. An increase in the rigor of the studies, driven by methodological improvements, should be a major priority in preclinical studies, thus reducing the ultimate translational failure. Yet, most of the clinical trials used autologous bone marrow mononuclear cells (BMCs), thereafter termed "first-generation stem cells" attracted by the claims of the potential and simplicity of BMCs (126); however, unselected BMCs, even though enriched in $CD34^+$ cells compared to PBMCs, may represent a cell product with limited potential for improving the clinical outcomes. For instance, the clinical success of primary percutaneous coronary interventions after acute myocardial infarction is so remarkable that demonstrating the efficacy of new cell therapies in those patients is challenging. A meta-analysis studied the safety and efficacy of intracoronary cell therapy after acute myocardial infarction in patients from 12 randomized trials: the cell therapy was observed to be safe and well tolerated by patients but provided no benefit in terms of clinical events or changes in the left ventricular function, as a surrogate endpoint [127]. In contrast, the application of cell therapy remains an open question in chronic heart failure and refractory angina [128]. To overcome these negative results, unfractioned BMCs could be replaced with cell products enriched for more potent cells, such as $CD34^+$ cells, which have been termed "second-generation stem cells" [84, 126]. However, even if autologous BMCs, either unfractioned or not, represented a possible source for cell therapy, in patients with metabolic diseases this would be a hindrance because they could be intrinsically defective. Indeed, prior studies have shown that diabetic HSPCs have an impaired angiogenic function and differentiation capacity (129), while a recent double-blind randomized controlled trial of bone marrow cell therapy for critical limb ischemia showed that the benefit was worse in patients with diabetes than in nondiabetic patients [129]. Therefore, it might be necessary to manipulate the cells *ex vivo* to improve their pro-angiogenic functions, and this will require the establishment of standardized assays to measure their potency. On the other hand, culturing and expanding endothelial progenitors, albeit possible, is challenging and still faces the possibility that cells might retain a certain degree of impairment, as per the phenomenon known as "hyperglycemic memory" [27]. A meta-analysis reviewed the safety and efficacy of studies performing autologous cell therapy for intractable peripheral arterial disease/critical limb ischemia, which is a life-threatening complication in patients with diabetes, for which amputation often represents the only option [130]. Overall, cell therapy was found to be safe and may have the potential to reduce the risk of major amputation (-36%) and improved the probability of wound healing (+59%). The sub-analyses showed that intramuscular injections may be preferable to intra-arterial infusion, due to the presence of significant stenotic leg arteries, and that mobilized PB-MNCs may outperform BMCs. This point is particularly relevant since patients with metabolic diseases are poor mobilizers [131]. Therefore, we were rather disappointed when patients with ischemic wounds treated with plerixafor, which induced a robust mobilization of HSPCs and endothelial progenitors, displayed no improvement in wound healing [121]. It is possible, as for peripheral arterial disease, that poor blood flow at the sites of wound healing compromised the recruitment of pro-angiogenic cells, as was indeed reported in the pre-clinical studies in mice [132]. This evidence suggests that the local administration of cell products is preferable to systemic injection, in order to increase the chance of vascular improvements. As shown for other cell therapies, multiple rounds of mobilization or repeated administration of endothelial progenitors could have a better impact on the clinical outcomes [133]. Moreover, we have recently shown that the same signaling pathway causing inflammatory myelopoiesis is also responsible for stem cell mobilopathy in diabetes [78]. It is possible that plerixafor may have mobilized anti-angiogenic or proinflammatory cells exerting detrimental effects on wound healing. Thus, mobilizing endothelial progenitors or HSPCs without countering myelopoiesis and metabolic alterations might be insufficient to improve the outcomes.

The goal of cell therapy in metabolic diseases is ultimately to improve the vascularization of ischemic and poorly perfused areas to avoid the loss of tissue function, or, possibly, to boost reparatory mechanisms to constrain endothelial dysfunction. The downside is that an excess of angiogenesis could be detrimental within certain clinical settings. During the natural history of atherosclerosis, the mobilization of endothelial progenitors could counteract their decline, preventing endothelial dysfunction, and possibly promoting plaque regression [134]. At the later stages, when the plaque develops a hypoxic necrotic core, endothelial progenitors might contribute to intraplaque neovascularization and vulnerability [135, 136]. Notably, a definitive role of endothelial progenitors for plaque homeostasis is still a matter of debate [137]. Diabetic retinopathy is often described as a diabetic paradox, because it is driven by an excess of angiogenesis. Some works associated a low count of endothelial progenitors to the development of retinopathy [59, 138], while other studies reported a positive correlation between the count and the function of endothelial progenitors and diabetic retinopathy [139-141]. However, whether an increase in the number and function of endothelial progenitors can fuel the progression of diabetic retinopathy is currently unknown; nevertheless, it should be carefully acknowledged as an undesired side effect of cell therapy. It is worth mentioning that the stimulation of pro-angiogenic cells could theoretically increase the risk of cancer development or dissemination, since individuals with diabetes have an increased susceptibility to some forms of cancer. This evidence recalls the importance and the difficulties of the selection of the patients to be treated with cell therapy: a higher degree of heterogeneity could potentially mask the effect of the therapy itself [121]. Indeed, those with an improved functional capacity after therapy might have had less severe vascular disease at baseline. Furthermore, the proper identification of high-risk patients and the choice between surrogate versus clinical endpoints, could mark the difference between trial failure or success [142].

At a point 15 years after the initial groundbreaking trials, the scientific community is still attracted to the potential of cell therapy for the treatment of high-risk patients with metabolic diseases; however, we now know how difficult this challenge has proven to be (Figure 2).

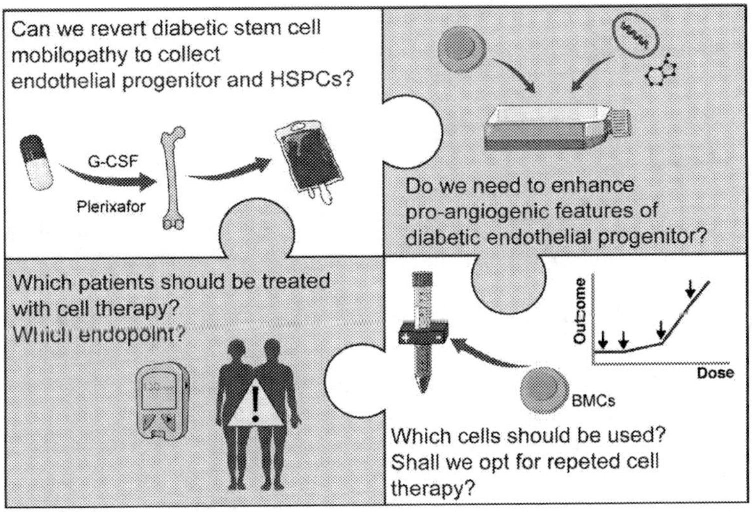

Figure 2. Unresolved questions on cell therapy for metabolic diseases. See the corresponding paragraph in the text for a discussion of the issues depicted in the figure. HSCPs, hematopoietic stem/progenitor cells. BMCs, bone marrow mononuclear cells. G-CSF, granulocyte colony stimulation factor.

Conclusion

The discovery of endothelial progenitors represented a milestone for research in the cardiovascular and metabolic field. Their definition might still be a work in progress and remains a challenge; however, they re-shaped the field by providing insights on the pivotal relationships between the vascular and hematopoietic systems. At the same time, the concepts of cardiovascular regeneration and the contribution of endothelial progenitors have dramatically improved since 1997, thanks to the technological developments that allowed a revision of the previous drawbacks in research findings and the establishment of a rigorous scrutiny. Moving forward, the field should study the mechanism of action of endothelial progenitors (particularly paracrine mechanisms) at the preclinical level and the possibility of combining cell therapy with acellular therapies, such as directly delivering siRNA to endothelial progenitors using nano-encapsulation or genome editing with CRISPR/Cas9 [143, 144]. This is particularly relevant for patients facing long-term metabolic diseases that ultimately will impact the function of endothelial progenitors and homeostasis of the bone marrow. While the application of endothelial progenitors for cell therapy is still far from reaching clinical practice, their measurement in patients with metabolic diseases can improve cardiovascular risk stratification, and ultimately their health span.

References

[1] Asahara T, Murohara T, Sullivan A, Silver M, Van Der Zee R, Li T, et al. Isolation of putative progenitor endothelial cells for angiogenesis. *Science* (80). 1997; 275 (5302):964–7.

[2] Pelosi E, Valtieri M, Coppola S, Botta R, Gabbianelli M, Lulli V, et al. Identification of the hemangioblast in postnatal life. *Blood.* 2002;100(9):3203–8.

[3] Case J, Mead LE, Bessler WK, Prater D, White HA, Saadatzadeh MR, et al. Human CD34+AC133+VEGFR-2+ cells are not endothelial progenitor cells but distinct, primitive hematopoietic progenitors. *Exp Hematol* [Internet]. 2007 Jul;35(7):1109–18. Available from: http://www.ncbi.nlm.nih.gov/pubmed/17588480.

[4] Yoder MC, Mead LE, Prater D, Krier TR, Mroueh KN, Li F, et al. Redefining endothelial progenitor cells via clonal analysis and hematopoietic stem/progenitor cell principals. *Blood.* 2007;109(5):1801–9.

[5] Lancrin C, Sroczynska P, Stephenson C, Allen T, Kouskoff V, Lacaud G. The haemangioblast generates haematopoietic cells through a haemogenic endothelium stage. *Nature*. 2009;457(7231):892–5.

[6] Feng T, Gao Z, Kou S, Huang X, Jiang Z, Lu Z, et al. No Evidence for Erythro-Myeloid Progenitor-Derived Vascular Endothelial Cells in Multiple Organs. *Circ Res* [Internet]. 2020;127(10):1221–32. Available from: http://www.ncbi.nlm.nih.gov/pubmed/32791884.

[7] Medina RJ, Barber CL, Sabatier F, Dignat-George F, Melero-Martin JM, Khosrotehrani K, et al. Endothelial Progenitors: A Consensus Statement on Nomenclature. *Stem Cells Transl Med* [Internet]. 2017 May;6(5):1316–20. Available from: https://onlinelibrary.wiley.com/doi/10.1002/sctm.16-0360.

[8] Peichev M, Naiyer AJ, Pereira D, Zhu Z, Lane WJ, Williams M, et al. Expression of VEGFR-2 and AC133 by circulating human CD34+ cells identifies a population of functional endothelial precursors. *Blood* [Internet]. 2000;95(3):952–8. Available from: http://www.ncbi.nlm.nih.gov/pubmed/10648408.
[9] Cines DB, Pollak ES, Buck CA, Loscalzo J, Zimmerman GA, McEver RP, et al. Endothelial cells in physiology and in the pathophysiology of vascular disorders. *Blood.* 1998;91(10):3527–61.
[10] Lorenzen JM, Dietrich B, Fiedler J, Jazbutyte V, Fleissner F, Karpinski N, et al. Pathologic endothelial response and impaired function of circulating angiogenic cells in patients with Fabry disease. *Basic Res Cardiol.* 2013;108(1).
[11] Madonna R, De Caterina R. Cellular and molecular mechanisms of vascular injury in diabetes - Part I: Pathways of vascular disease in diabetes. *Vascul Pharmacol* [Internet]. 2011;54(3–6):68–74. Available from: http://dx.doi.org/10.1016/j.vph.2011.03.005.
[12] Seshasai SRK, Kaptoge S, Thompson A, Di Angelantonio E, Gao P, Sarwar N, et al. Diabetes mellitus, fasting glucose, and risk of cause-specific death. *N Engl J Med* [Internet]. 2011 Mar 3;364(9):829–41. Available from: http://www.ncbi.nlm.nih.gov/pubmed/21366474.
[13] Fadini GP, Morieri ML, Boscari F, Fioretto P, Maran A, Busetto L, et al. Newly-diagnosed diabetes and admission hyperglycemia predict COVID-19 severity by aggravating respiratory deterioration. *Diabetes Res Clin Pract* [Internet]. 2020 Oct;168:108374. Available from: http://www.ncbi.nlm.nih.gov/pubmed/32805345.
[14] Khan MAB, Hashim MJ, King JK, Govender RD, Mustafa H, Kaabi J Al. Epidemiology of Type 2 diabetes - Global burden of disease and forecasted trends. *J Epidemiol Glob Health.* 2020;10(1):107–11.
[15] Deedwania PC. Diabetes is a vascular disease: The role of endothelial dysfunction in pathophysiology of cardiovascular disease in diabetes. *Cardiol Clin.* 2004;22(4):505–9.
[16] Shah MS, Brownlee M. Molecular and cellular mechanisms of cardiovascular disorders in diabetes. *Circ Res*. 2016;118(11):1808–29.
[17] Brownlee M. The pathobiology of diabetic complications: a unifying mechanism. *Diabetes* [Internet]. 2005 Jun;54(6):1615–25. Available from: http://www.ncbi.nlm.nih.gov/pubmed/15919781.
[18] Avogaro A, Albiero M, Menegazzo L, De Kreutzenberg S, Fadini GPGP. Endothelial dysfunction in diabetes: The role of reparatory mechanisms. *Diabetes* Care. 2011 May;34(SUPPL. 2):S285-90.
[19] Loomans CJM, de Koning EJP, Staal FJT, Rookmaaker MB, Verseyden C, de Boer HC, et al. Endothelial Progenitor Cell Dysfunction: A novel concept in the pathogenesis of vascular complications of type 1 diabetes. *Diabetes* [Internet]. 2004 Jan 1;53(1):195–9. Available from: http://diabetes.diabetesjournals.org/cgi/doi/10.2337/diabetes.53.1.195.
[20] Tepper OM, Galiano RD, Capla JM, Kalka C, Gagne PJ, Jacobowitz GR, et al. Human endothelial progenitor cells from type II diabetics exhibit impaired proliferation, adhesion, and incorporation into vascular structures. *Circulation*

[Internet]. 2002 Nov 26;106(22):2781–6. Available from: https://www.ahajournals.org/doi/10.1161/01.CIR.0000039526.42991.93.

[21] Fadini GP, Coracina A, Baesso I, Agostini C, Tiengo A, Avogaro A, et al. Peripheral blood CD34+KDR+ endothelial progenitor cells are determinants of subclinical atherosclerosis in a middle-aged general population. *Stroke.* 2006; 37(9):2277–82.

[22] Fadini GPGP, Sartore S, Albiero M, Baesso I, Murphy E, Menegolo M, et al. Number and function of endothelial progenitor cells as a marker of severity for diabetic vasculopathy. *Arterioscler Thromb Vasc Biol.* 2006 Sep;26(9):2140–6.

[23] Fadini GP, Miorin M, Facco M, Bonamico S, Baesso I, Grego F, et al. Circulating endothelial progenitor cells are reduced in peripheral vascular complications of type 2 diabetes mellitus. *J Am Coll Cardiol.* 2005;45(9):1449–57.

[24] Tobler K, Freudenthaler A, Baumgartner-Parzer SM, Wolzt M, Ludvik B, Nansalmaa E, et al. Reduction of both number and proliferative activity of human endothelial progenitor cells in obesity. *Int J Obes.* 2010;34(4):687–700.

[25] Heida NM, Müller JP, Cheng IF, Leifheit-Nestler M, Faustin V, Riggert J, et al. Effects of Obesity and Weight Loss on the Functional Properties of Early Outgrowth Endothelial Progenitor Cells. *J Am Coll Cardiol.* 2010;55(4):357–67.

[26] Müller-Ehmsen J, Braun D, Schneider T, Pfister R, Worm N, Wielckens K, et al. Decreased number of circulating progenitor cells in obesity: Beneficial effects of weight reduction. *Eur Heart J.* 2008;29(12):1560–8.

[27] Giacco F, Brownlee M. Oxidative stress and diabetic complications. *Circ Res.* 2010;107(9):1058–70.

[28] Asahara T, Masuda H, Takahashi T, Kalka C, Pastore C, Silver M, et al. Bone marrow origin of endothelial progenitor cells responsible for postnatal vasculogenesis in physiological and pathological neovascularization. *Circ Res* [Internet]. 1999 Aug 6;85(3):221–8. Available from: http://www.ncbi.nlm.nih.gov/ pubmed/ 10436164.

[29] Fadini GP, de Kreutzenberg S V. Mariano V, Boscaro E, Bertolini F, Mancuso P, et al. Optimized glycaemic control achieved with add-on basal insulin therapy improves indexes of endothelial damage and regeneration in type 2 diabetic patients with macroangiopathy: A randomized crossover trial comparing detemir versus glargine. *Diabetes, Obes Metab.* 2011;13(8):718–25.

[30] Fadini GP, Boscaro E, De Kreutzenberg S, Agostini C, Seeger F, Dimmeler S, et al. Time course and mechanisms of circulating progenitor cell reduction in the natural history of type 2 diabetes. *Diabetes Care.* 2010;33(5):1097–102.

[31] Di Stefano V, Cencioni C, Zaccagnini G, Magenta A, Capogrossi MC, Martelli F. P66ShcA modulates oxidative stress and survival of endothelial progenitor cells in response to high glucose. *Cardiovasc Res.* 2009;82(3):421–9.

[32] Giorgio M, Migliaccio E, Orsini F, Paolucci D, Moroni M, Contursi C, et al. Electron transfer between cytochrome c and p66Shc generates reactive oxygen species that trigger mitochondrial apoptosis. *Cell.* 2005;122(2):221–33.

[33] Chen YLYH, Lin SJ, Lin FY, Wu TC, Tsao CR, Huang PH, et al. High glucose impairs early and late endothelial progenitor cells by modifying nitric oxide-related but not oxidative stress-mediated mechanisms. *Diabetes.* 2007;56(6):1559–68.

[34] Camici GG, Schiavoni M, Francia P, Bachschmid M, Martin-Padura I, Hersberger M, et al. Genetic deletion of p66Shc adaptor protein prevents hyperglycemia-induced endothelial dysfunction and oxidative stress. *Proc Natl Acad Sci USA* [Internet]. 2007;104(12):5217–22. Available from: http://www.pnas.org/cgi/doi/10.1073/pnas.0609656104.

[35] Paneni F, Mocharla P, Akhmedov A, Costantino S, Osto E, Volpe M, et al. Gene silencing of the mitochondrial adaptor p66Shc suppresses vascular hyperglycemic memory in diabetes. *Circ Res.* 2012;111(3):278–89.

[36] Pagnin E, Fadini G, De Toni R, Tiengo A, Calò L, Avogaro A. Diabetes induces p66shc gene expression in human peripheral blood mononuclear cells: Relationship to oxidative. *J Clin Endocrinol Metab* [Internet]. 2005;90(2):1130–6. Available from: https://academic.oup.com/jcem/article-lookup/doi/10.1210/jc.2004-1283.

[37] Zhang Y, Herbert B, Rajashekhar G, Ingram DA, Yoder MC, Clauss M, et al. Premature senescence of highly proliferative endothelial progenitor cells is induced by tumor necrosis factor-α via the p38 mitogen-activated protein kinase pathway . *FASEB J.* 2009;23(5):1358–65.

[38] Seeger FH, Haendeler J, Walter DH, Rochwalsky U, Reinhold J, Urbich C, et al. P38 Mitogen-Activated Protein Kinase Downregulates Endothelial Progenitor Cells. *Circulation.* 2005;111(9):1184–91.

[39] Loomans CJM, Van Haperen R, Duijs JM, Verseyden C, De Crom R, Leenen PJM, et al. Differentiation of bone marrow-derived endothelial progenitor cells is shifted into a proinflammatory phenotype by hyperglycemia. *Mol Med* [Internet]. 2009;15(5–6):152–9. Available from: http://www.molmed.org/content/pdfstore/152_159.vanZonneveld.00032.PDF.

[40] Hazra S, Jarajapu YPR, Stepps V, Caballero S, Thinschmidt JS, Sautina L, et al. Long-term type 1 diabetes influences haematopoietic stem cells by reducing vascular repair potential and increasing inflammatory monocyte generation in a murine model. *Diabetologia*. 2013;56(3):644–53.

[41] Speer T, Rohrer L, Blyszczuk P, Shroff R, Kuschnerus K, Kränkel N, et al. Abnormal high-density lipoprotein induces endothelial dysfunction via activation of toll-like receptor-2. *Immunity.* 2013;38(4):754–68.

[42] Spigoni V, Fantuzzi F, Fontana A, Cito M, Derlindati E, Zavaroni I, et al. Stearic acid at physiologic concentrations induces in vitro lipotoxicity in circulating angiogenic cells. *Atherosclerosis* [Internet]. 2017;265:162–71. Available from: https://doi.org/10.1016/j.atherosclerosis.2017.09.004.

[43] Pirro M, Bagaglia F, Paoletti L, Razzi R, Mannarino MR. Hypercholesterolemia-associated endothelial progenitor cell dysfunction. *Ther Adv Cardiovasc Dis.* 2008; 2(5):329–39.

[44] Imanishi T, Hano T, Sawamura T, Nishio I. Oxidized low-density lipoprotein induces endothelial progenitor cell senescence, leading to cellular dysfunction. *Clin Exp Pharmacol Physiol*. 2004;31(7):407–13.

[45] Wu Y, Wang Q, Cheng L, Wang J, Lu G. Effect of oxidized low-density lipoprotein on survival and function of endothelial progenitor cell mediated by p38 signal pathway. *J Cardiovasc Pharmacol.* 2009;53(2):151–6.

[46] Ma FX, Zhou B, Chen Z, Ren Q, Lu SH, Sawamura T, et al. Oxidized low density lipoprotein impairs endothelial progenitor cells by regulation of endothelial nitric oxide synthase. *J Lipid Res* [Internet]. 2006 Jun;47(6):1227–37. Available from: http://www.ncbi.nlm.nih.gov/pubmed/16522925.

[47] Vasa M, Fichtlscherer S, Aicher A, Adler K, Urbich C, Martin H, et al. Number and migratory activity of circulating endothelial progenitor cells inversely correlate with risk factors for coronary artery disease. *Circ Res* [Internet]. 2001;89(1):E1-7. Available from: http://circres.ahajournals.org/cgi/doi/10.1161/hh1301.093953.

[48] Noor R, Shuaib U, Wang CX, Todd K, Ghani U, Schwindt B, et al. High-density lipoprotein cholesterol regulates endothelial progenitor cells by increasing eNOS and preventing apoptosis. *Atherosclerosis.* 2007;192(1):92–9.

[49] Rossi F, Bertone C, Montanile F, Miglietta F, Lubrano C, Gandini L, et al. HDL cholesterol is a strong determinant of endothelial progenitor cells in hypercholesterolemic subjects. *Microvasc Res* [Internet]. 2010 Sep;80(2):274–9. Available from: http://dx.doi.org/10.1016/j.mvr.2010.05.003.

[50] Avogaro A, Fadini GP, Gallo A, Pagnin E, De Kreutzenberg S. Endothelial dysfunction in type 2 diabetes mellitus. *Nutr Metab Cardiovasc Dis.* 2006;16 (SUPPL. 1):S39-45.

[51] Fadini GPGP, Albiero M, Seeger F, Poncina N, Menegazzo L, Angelini A, et al. Stem cell compartmentalization in diabetes and high cardiovascular risk reveals the role of DPP-4 in diabetic stem cell mobilopathy. *Basic Res Cardiol.* 2013 Jan; 108(1):1–12.

[52] Fadini GP, Losordo D, Dimmeler S. Critical reevaluation of endothelial progenitor cell phenotypes for therapeutic and diagnostic use. *Circ Res.* 2012;110(4):624–37.

[53] Fadini GPP, Sartore S, Schiavon M, Albiero M, Baesso I, Cabrelle A, et al. Diabetes impairs progenitor cell mobilisation after hindlimb ischaemia-reperfusion injury in rats. *Diabetologia.* 2006 Dec;49(12):3075–84.

[54] Ceradini DJ, Kulkarni AR, Callaghan MJ, Tepper OM, Bastidas N, Kleinman ME, et al. Progenitor cell trafficking is regulated by hypoxic gradients through HIF-1 induction of SDF-1. *Nat Med* [Internet]. 2004 Aug;10(8):858–64. Available from: http://www.ncbi.nlm.nih.gov/pubmed/15235597.

[55] Ceradini DJ, Yao D, Grogan RH, Callaghan MJ, Edelstein D, Brownlee M, et al. Decreasing intracellular superoxide corrects defective ischemia-induced new vessel formation in diabetic mice. *J Biol Chem.* 2008;283(16):10930–8.

[56] Murohara T, Asahara T, Silver M, Bauters C, Masuda H, Kalka C, et al. Nitric oxide synthase modulates angiogenesis in response to tissue ischemia. *J Clin Invest.* 1998;101(11):2567–78.

[57] Aicher A, Heeschen C, Mildner-Rihm C, Urbich C, Ihling C, Technau-Ihling K, et al. Essential role of endothelial nitric oxide synthase for mobilization of stem and progenitor cells. *Nat Med* [Internet]. 2003 Nov;9(11):1370–6. Available from: http://www.ncbi.nlm.nih.gov/pubmed/14556003.

[58] Gallagher KA, Liu Z-J, Xiao M, Chen H, Goldstein LJ, Buerk DG, et al. Diabetic impairments in NO-mediated endothelial progenitor cell mobilization and homing are reversed by hyperoxia and SDF-1 alpha. *J Clin Invest* [Internet]. 2007

May;117(5):1249–59. Available from: http://www.ncbi.nlm.nih.gov/pubmed/1747 6357.

[59] Busik J V. Tikhonenko M, Bhatwadekar A, Opreanu M, Yakubova N, Caballero S, et al. Diabetic retinopathy is associated with bone marrow neuropathy and a depressed peripheral clock. *J Exp Med* [Internet]. 2009;206(13):2897–906. Available from: http://www.jem.org/lookup/doi/10.1084/jem.20090889.

[60] Oikawa A, Siragusa M, Quaini F, Mangialardi G, Katare RG, Caporali A, et al. Diabetes mellitus induces bone marrow microangiopathy. *Arterioscler Thromb Vasc Biol* [Internet]. 2010 Mar 1;30(3):498–508. Available from: http://atvb.aha journals.org/cgi/doi/10.1161/ATVBAHA.109.200154.

[61] Januszyk M, Sorkin M, Glotzbach JP, Vial IN, Maan ZN, Rennert RC, et al. Diabetes irreversibly depletes bone marrow-derived mesenchymal progenitor cell subpopulations. *Diabetes.* 2014;63(9):3047–56.

[62] Morrison SJ, Scadden DT. The bone marrow niche for haematopoietic stem cells. *Nature*. 2014;505(7483):327–34.

[63] Albiero M, Poncina N, Tjwa M, Ciciliot S, Menegazzo L, Ceolotto G, et al. Diabetes causes bone marrow autonomic neuropathy and impairs stem cell mobilization via dysregulated p66Shc and Sirt1. *Diabetes* [Internet]. 2014 Apr 1;63(4):1353–65. Available from: http://diabetes.diabetesjournals.org/cgi/doi/10.2 337/db13-0894.

[64] Albiero M, D'Anna M, Bonora BM, Zuccolotto G, Rosato A, Giorgio M, et al. Hematopoietic and non-hematopoietic p66Shc differentially regulates stem cell traffic and vascular response to ischemia in diabetes. *Antioxid Redox Signal* [Internet]. 2021 Sep 20; Available from: http://www.ncbi.nlm.nih.gov/pubmed/ 34538132.

[65] Lévesque J-P, Purton LE, Hidalgo A, Zon LI, Katayama Y, Scadden DT, et al. In memory of Paul Sylvain Frenette, a pioneering explorer of the hematopoietic stem cell niche who left far too early. *Exp Hematol* [Internet]. 2021 Aug 14; Available from: http://www.ncbi.nlm.nih.gov/pubmed/34403758.

[66] Katayama Y, Battista M, Kao WM, Hidalgo A, Peired AJ, Thomas SA, et al. Signals from the sympathetic nervous system regulate hematopoietic stem cell egress from bone marrow. *Cell* [Internet]. 2006 Jan;124(2):407–21. Available from: http://linkinghub.elsevier.com/retrieve/pii/S0092867405013280.

[67] Ferraro F, Lymperi S, Méndez-Ferrer S, Saez B, Spencer JA, Yeap BY, et al. Diabetes impairs hematopoietic stem cell mobilization by altering niche function. *Sci Transl Med* [Internet]. 2011 Oct 12;3(104):104ra101-104ra101. Available from: http://stm.sciencemag.org/cgi/doi/10.1126/scitranslmed.3002191.

[68] DiPersio JF. Diabetic stem-cell "mobilopathy." *N Engl J Med* [Internet]. 2011 Dec 29;365(26):2536–8. Available from: http://www.ncbi.nlm.nih.gov/pubmed/22204 729.

[69] Fadini GP. Is bone marrow another target of diabetic complications? *Eur J Clin Invest* [Internet]. 2011 Apr;41(4):457–63. Available from: http://www.ncbi.nlm. nih.gov/pubmed/21175550.

[70] Spinetti G, Cordella D, Fortunato O, Sangalli E, Losa S, Gotti A, et al. Global remodeling of the vascular stem cell niche in bone marrow of diabetic patients:

Implication of the microRNA-155/FOXO3a signaling pathway. *Circ Res* [Internet]. 2013 Feb 1;112(3):510–22. Available from: http://circres.ahajournals.org/lookup/doi/10.1161/CIRCRESAHA.112.300598.

[71] Fadini GPGP, Albiero M, De Kreutzenberg SVSV, Boscaro E, Cappellari R, Marescotti M, et al. Diabetes impairs stem cell and proangiogenic cell mobilization in humans. *Diabetes Care* [Internet]. 2013 Apr;36(4):943–9. Available from: http://www.pubmedcentral.nih.gov/articlerender.fcgi?artid=PMC4589553.

[72] Petit I, Ponomaryov T, Zipori D, Tsvee L. G-CSF induces stem cell mobilization by decreasing bone marrow SDF-1 and up-regulating CXCR4. *Nat Immunol.* 2002; 3(7):687–94.

[73] Christopherson KW, Cooper S, Hangoc G, Broxmeyer HE. CD26 is essential for normal G-CSF–induced progenitor cell mobilization as determined by CD26−/− mice. *Exp Hematol* [Internet]. 2003 Nov;31(11):1126–34. Available from: http://www.ncbi.nlm.nih.gov/pubmed/14585379.

[74] Fadini GPGP, Fiala M, Cappellari R, Danna M, Park S, Poncina N, et al. Diabetes limits stem cell mobilization following G-CSF but not plerixafor. *Diabetes.* 2015 Aug;64(8):2969–77.

[75] Chow A, Lucas D, Hidalgo A, Méndez-Ferrer S, Hashimoto D, Scheiermann C, et al. Bone marrow CD169+ macrophages promote the retention of hematopoietic stem and progenitor cells in the mesenchymal stem cell niche. *J Exp Med* [Internet]. 2011;208(2):761–71. Available from: http://www.jem.org/lookup/doi/10.1084/jem.20101688.

[76] Albiero M, Poncina N, Ciciliot S, Cappellari R, Menegazzo L, Ferraro F, et al. Bone Marrow Macrophages Contribute to Diabetic Stem Cell Mobilopathy by Producing Oncostatin M. *Diabetes* [Internet]. 2015 Aug;64(8):2957–68. Available from: http://diabetes.diabetesjournals.org/lookup/doi/10.2337/db14-1473.

[77] Nagareddy PR, Murphy AJ, Stirzaker RA, Hu Y, Yu S, Miller RG, et al. Hyperglycemia promotes myelopoiesis and impairs the resolution of atherosclerosis. Cell Metab [Internet]. 2013 May;17(5):695–708. Available from: http://linkinghub.elsevier.com/retrieve/pii/S1550413113001435.

[78] Albiero M, Ciciliot S, Tedesco S, Menegazzo L, D'Anna M, Scattolini V, et al. Diabetes-Associated Myelopoiesis Drives Stem Cell Mobilopathy Through an OSM-p66Shc Signaling Pathway. *Diabetes* [Internet]. 2019 Jun 1;68(6):1303– 14. Available from: http://diabetes.diabetesjournals.org/lookup/doi/10.2337/db19-0080.

[79] Albiero M, Tedesco S, Amendolagine FI, D'Anna M, Migliozzi L, Zuccolotto G, et al. Inhibition of SGLT-2 rescues bone marrow cell traffic for vascular repair. Role of glucose control and ketogenesis. *Diabetes* [Internet]. 2021 Apr 26; Available from: http://www.ncbi.nlm.nih.gov/pubmed/33903150.

[80] Vasam G, Joshi S, Jarajapu YPR. Impaired Mobilization of Vascular Reparative Bone Marrow Cells in Streptozotocin-Induced Diabetes but not in Leptin Receptor-Deficient db/db Mice. *Sci Rep* [Internet]. 2016 Sep 18;6(1):26131. Available from: http://dx.doi.org/10.1038/srep26131.

[81] Fujisawa T, Tura-Ceide O, Hunter A, Mitchell A, Vesey A, Medine C, et al. Endothelial progenitor cells do not originate from the bone marrow. *Circulation.* 2019;140(18):1524–6.

[82] Strimbu K, Tavel JA. What are biomarkers? *Curr Opin HIV AIDS*. 2010;5(6):463–6.

[83] Zethelius B, Berglund L, Sundström J, Ingelsson E, Basu S, Larsson A, et al. Use of Multiple Biomarkers to Improve the Prediction of Death from Cardiovascular Causes. *N Engl J Med.* 2008;358(20):2107–16.

[84] Kawamoto A, Iwasaki H, Kusano K, Murayama T, Oyamada A, Silver M, et al. CD34-positive cells exhibit increased potency and safety for therapeutic neovascularization after myocardial infarction compared with total mononuclear cells. *Circulation* [Internet]. 2006 Nov 14;114(20):2163–9. Available from: http://www.ncbi.nlm.nih.gov/pubmed/17075009.

[85] Madeddu P, Emanueli C, Pelosi E, Salis MB, Cerio AM, Bonanno G, et al. Transplantation of low dose CD34 + Kdr + cells promotes vascular and muscular regeneration in ischemic limbs . *FASEB J* [Internet]. 2004;18(14):1737–9. Available from: http://www.fasebj.org/cgi/doi/10.1096/fj.04-2192fje.

[86] Patel RS, Li Q, Ghasemzadeh N, Eapen DJ, Moss LD, Janjua AU, et al. Circulating CD34+ progenitor cells and risk of mortality in a population with coronary artery disease. *Circ Res*. 2015;116(2):289–97.

[87] Werner N, Kosiol S, Schiegl T, Ahlers P, Walenta K, Link A, et al. Circulating endothelial progenitor cells and cardiovascular outcomes. *N Engl J Med* [Internet]. 2005;353(10):999–1007. Available from: http://www.nejm.org/doi/abs/10.1056/NEJMoa043814.

[88] Fadini GP, Maruyama S, Ozaki T, Taguchi A, Meigs J, Dimmeler S, et al. Circulating progenitor cell count for cardiovascular risk stratification: A pooled analysis. *PLoS One*. 2010;5(7):e11488.

[89] Fadini GP, Agostini C, Boscaro E, Avogaro A. Mechanisms and significance of progenitor cell reduction in the metabolic syndrome. *Metab Syndr Relat Disord.* 2009;7(1):5–10.

[90] Fadini GP, De Kreutzenberg SV, Coracina A, Baesso I, Agostini C, Tiengo A, et al. Circulating CD34+ cells, metabolic syndrome, and cardiovascular risk. *Eur Heart J*. 2006;27(18):2247–55.

[91] Rigato M, Avogaro A, Fadini GP. Levels of Circulating Progenitor Cells, Cardiovascular Outcomes and Death: A Meta-Analysis of Prospective Observational Studies. *Circ Res* [Internet]. 2016 Jun 10;118(12):1930–9. Available from: http://www.ncbi.nlm.nih.gov/pubmed/27073015.

[92] Pozzoli O, Vella P, Iaffaldano G, Parente V, Devanna P, Lacovich M, et al. Endothelial fate and angiogenic properties of human CD34+ progenitor cells in zebrafish. *Arterioscler Thromb Vasc Biol.* 2011;31(7):1589–97.

[93] Hernandez SL, Gong JH, Chen L, Wu IH, Sun JK, Keenan HA, et al. Characterization of circulating and endothelial progenitor cells in patients with extreme-duration type 1 diabetes. *Diabetes Care* [Internet]. 2014;37(8):2193–201. Available from: http://care.diabetesjournals.org/lookup/doi/10.2337/dc13-2547

[94] Sarto P, Balducci E, Balconi G, Fiordaliso F, Merlo L, Tuzzato G, et al. Effects of Exercise Training on Endothelial Progenitor Cells in Patients With Chronic Heart Failure. *J Card Fail.* 2007;13(9):701–8.

[95] Ross MD. Endothelial Regenerative Capacity and Aging: Influence of Diet, Exercise and Obesity. *Curr Cardiol Rev.* 2018;14(4):233–44.

[96] Avogaro A. Insulin resistance: trigger or concomitant factor in the metabolic syndrome. *Panminerva Med* [Internet]. 2006 Mar;48(1):3–12. Available from: http://www.ncbi.nlm.nih.gov/pubmed/16633326.

[97] Albiero M, Fadini GPP. Pharmacologic targeting of the diabetic stem cell mobilopathy. *Pharmacol Res* [Internet]. 2018 Sep;135:18–24. Available from: http://www.ncbi.nlm.nih.gov/pubmed/30030170.

[98] Dama A, Baggio C, Boscaro C, Albiero M, Cignarella A. Estrogen Receptor Functions and Pathways at the Vascular Immune Interface. *Int J Mol Sci* [Internet]. 2021 Apr 20;22(8). Available from: http://www.ncbi.nlm.nih.gov/pubmed/33923 905.

[99] Albiero M, Menegazzo L, Avogaro A, Fadini GPGP. Pharmacologic Targeting of Endothelial Progenitor Cells. *Cardiovasc Hematol Disord Targets*. 2010 Mar;10 (1):16–32.

[100] Dimmeler S, Fleming I, Fisslthaler B, Hermann C, Busse R, Zeiher AM. Activation of nitric oxide synthase in endothelial cells by Akt- dependent phosphorylation. *Nature* [Internet]. 1999;399(6736):601–5. Available from: http://www.nature.com/doifinder/10.1038/21224.

[101] Kureishi Y, Luo Z, Shiojima I, Bialik A, Fulton D, Lefer DJ, et al. The HMG-CoA reductase inhibitor simvastatin activates the protein kinase Akt and promotes angiogenesis in normocholesterolemic animals. *Nat Med* [Internet]. 2000 Sep; 6(9):1004–10. Available from: http://www.ncbi.nlm.nih.gov/pubmed/109733 20.

[102] Llevadot J, Murasawa S, Kureishi Y, Uchida S, Masuda H, Kawamoto A, et al. HMG-CoA reductase inhibitor mobilizes bone marrow–derived endothelial progenitor cells. *J Clin Invest* [Internet]. 2001;108(3):399–405. Available from: http://www.jci.org/cgi/content/abstract/108/3/399.

[103] Vasa M, Fichtlscherer S, Adler K, Aicher A, Martin H, Zeiher AM, et al. Increase in circulating endothelial progenitor cells by statin therapy in patients with stable coronary artery disease. *Circulation.* 2001;103(24):2885–90.

[104] Dimmeler S, Aicher A, Vasa M, Mildner-Rihm C, Adler K, Tiemann M, et al. HMG-CoA reductase inhibitors (statins) increase endothelial progenitor cells via the PI 3-kinase/Akt pathway. *J Clin Invest* [Internet]. 2001 Aug;108(3):391–7. Available from: http://www.ncbi.nlm.nih.gov/pubmed/11489932.

[105] Spyridopoulos I, Haendeler J, Urbich C, Brummendorf TH, Oh H, Schneider MD, et al. Statins enhance migratory capacity by upregulation of the telomere repeat-binding factor TRF2 in endothelial progenitor cells. *Circulation.* 2004;110(19): 3136–42.

[106] Ii M, Losordo DW. Statins and the endothelium. *Vascul Pharmacol.* 2007;46(1):1–9.

[107] Walter DH, Rittig K, Bahlmann FH, Kirchmair R, Silver M, Murayama T, et al. Statin therapy accelerates reendothelialization: A novel effect involving mobil-

ization and incorporation of bone marrow-derived endothelial progenitor cells. *Circulation.* 2002;105(25):3017–24.
[108] Fadini GP, de Kreutzenberg S V. Mariano V, Boscaro E, Bertolini F, Mancuso P, et al. Optimized glycaemic control achieved with add-on basal insulin therapy improves indexes of endothelial damage and regeneration in type 2 diabetic patients with macroangiopathy: a randomized crossover trial comparing detemir versus glargine. *Diabetes, Obes Meta*b [Internet]. 2011 Aug;13(8):718–25. Available from: https://onlinelibrary.wiley.com/doi/10.1111/j.1463-1326.2011.01396.x.
[109] Albiero M, Bonora BM, Fadini GP. Diabetes pharmacotherapy and circulating stem/progenitor cells. State of the art and evidence gaps. *Curr Opin Pharmacol* [Internet]. 2020 Dec;55:151–6. Available from: https://linkinghub.elsevier.com/retrieve/pii/S1471489220301259.
[110] Fadini GP, Avogaro A. Cardiovascular effects of DPP-4 inhibition: Beyond GLP-1. *Vascul Pharmacol* [Internet]. 2011;55(1–3):10–6. Available from: http://dx.doi.org/10.1016/j.vph.2011.05.001.
[111] Fadini GPGP, Boscaro E, Albiero M, Menegazzo L, Frison V, De Kreutzenberg S, et al. The oral dipeptidyl peptidase-4 inhibitor sitagliptin increases circulating endothelial progenitor cells in patients with type 2 diabetes: Possible role of stromal-derived factor-1α. *Diabetes Care.* 2010;33(7):1607–9.
[112] Nakamura K, Oe H, Kihara H, Shimada K, Fukuda S, Watanabe K, et al. DPP-4 inhibitor and alpha-glucosidase inhibitor equally improve endothelial function in patients with type 2 diabetes: EDGE study. *Cardiovasc Diabetol*. 2014;13(1):1–10.
[113] Dei Cas A, Spigoni V, Cito M, Aldigeri R, Ridolfi V, Marchesi E, et al. Vildagliptin, but not glibenclamide, increases circulating endothelial progenitor cell number: A 12-month randomized controlled trial in patients with type 2 diabetes. *Cardiovasc Diabetol.* 2017;16(1):1–11.
[114] Fadini GPGP, Bonora BMBM, Cappellari R, Menegazzo L, Vedovato M, Iori E, et al. Acute effects of linagliptin on progenitor cells, monocyte phenotypes, and soluble mediators in type 2 diabetes. *J Clin Endocrinol Metab* [Internet]. 2016 Feb;101(2):748–56. Available from: https://academic.oup.com/jcem/article-lookup/doi/10.1210/jc.2015-3716.
[115] Singh P, Hoggatt J, Kamocka MM, Mohammad KS, Saunders MR, Li H, et al. Neuropeptide Y regulates a vascular gateway for hematopoietic stem and progenitor cells. *J Clin Invest*. 2017;127(12):4527–40.
[116] Poncina N, Albiero M, Menegazzo L, Cappellari R, Avogaro A, Fadini GPGP. The dipeptidyl peptidase-4 inhibitor Saxagliptin improves function of circulating pro-angiogenic cells from type 2 diabetic patients. *Cardiovasc Diabetol.* 2014;13(1):1–16.
[117] Bonora BM, Cappellari R, Albiero M, Avogaro A, Fadini GP. Effects of SGLT2 Inhibitors on Circulating Stem and Progenitor Cells in Patients With Type 2 Diabetes. *J Clin Endocrinol Metab* [Internet]. 2018 Oct 1;103(10):3773–82. Available from: http://www.ncbi.nlm.nih.gov/pubmed/30113651.
[118] Hess DA, Terenzi DC, Verma S. SGLT-2 Inhibitors and Regenerative Cell Exhaustion. *Cell Metab* [Internet]. 2020 May;31(5):884–5. Available from: https://linkinghub.elsevier.com/retrieve/pii/S1550413120301856.

[119] Tedesco S, Ciciliot S, Menegazzo L, D'Anna M, Scattolini V, Cappellari R, et al. Pharmacologic PPAR-γ Activation Reprograms Bone Marrow Macrophages and Partially Rescues HSPC Mobilization in Human and Murine Diabetes. *Diabetes* [Internet]. 2020 Apr 28;69(7):1562–72. Available from: http://www.ncbi.nlm.nih.gov/pubmed/32345753.

[120] Nishimura Y, Ii M, Qin G, Hamada H, Asai J, Takenaka H, et al. CXCR4 antagonist AMD3100 accelerates impaired wound healing in diabetic mice. *J Invest Dermatol* [Internet]. 2012;132(3):711–20. Available from: http://dx.doi.org/10.1038/jid.2011.356.

[121] Bonora BM, Cappellari R, Mazzucato M, Rigato M, Grasso M, Menegolo M, et al. Stem cell mobilization with plerixafor and healing of diabetic ischemic wounds: A phase IIa, randomized, double-blind, placebo-controlled trial. *Stem Cells Transl Med.* 2020;9(9):965–73.

[122] Vågesjö E, Öhnstedt E, Mortier A, Lofton H, Huss F, Proost P, et al. Accelerated wound healing in mice by on-site production and delivery of CXCL12 by transformed lactic acid bacteria. *Proc Natl Acad Sci USA*. 2018;115(8):1895–900.

[123] Rota M, Kajstura J, Hosoda T, Bearzi C, Vitale S, Esposito G, et al. Bone marrow cells adopt the cardiomyogenic fate in vivo. *Proc Natl Acad Sci* [Internet]. 2007 Nov 6;104(45):17783–8. Available from: http://www.pnas.org/cgi/doi/10.1073/pnas.0706406104.

[124] Orlic D, Kajstura J, Chimenti S, Jakoniuk I, Anderson SM, Li B, et al. Bone marrow cells regenerate infarcted myocardium. *Nature* [Internet]. 2001 Apr 5;410(6829):701–5. Available from: http://www.ncbi.nlm.nih.gov/pubmed/11287958.

[125] Balsam LB, Wagers AJ, Christensen JL, Kofidis T, Weissmann IL, Robbins RC. Haematopoietic stem cells adopt mature haematopoietic fates in ischaemic myocardium. *Nature.* 2004;428(6983):668–73.

[126] Fanaroff AC, Morrow V, Krucoff MW, Seltzer JH, Perin EC, Taylor DA, et al. A path forward for regenerative medicine navigating regulatory challenges: Summary of findings from the cardiac safety research consortium/Texas heart institute international symposium on cardiovascular regenerative medicine. *Circ Res.* 2018; 123(4):495–505.

[127] Gyöngyösi M, Wojakowski W, Lemarchand P, Lunde K, Tendera M, Bartunek J, et al. Meta-analysis of cell-based CaRdiac stUdiEs (ACCRUE) in patients with acute myocardial infarction based on individual patient data. *Circ Res.* 2015; 116(8):1346–60.

[128] Bolli R. Cell therapy for acutemyocardial infarction: Requiescat in Pace. *Eur Heart J.* 2020;41(38):3711–4.

[129] Caballero S, Sengupta N, Afzal A, Chang K-H, Li Calzi S, Guberski DL, et al. Ischemic vascular damage can be repaired by healthy, but not diabetic, endothelial progenitor cells. *Diabetes* [Internet]. 2007 Apr;56(4):960–7. Available from: http://www.ncbi.nlm.nih.gov/pubmed/17395742.

[130] Rigato M, Monami M, Fadini GP. Autologous Cell Therapy for Peripheral Arterial Disease: Systematic Review and Meta-Analysis of Randomized, Nonrandomized,

and Noncontrolled Studies. *Circ Res* [Internet]. 2017 Apr 14;120(8):1326–40. Available from: http://www.ncbi.nlm.nih.gov/pubmed/28096194.

[131] Fadini GP, DiPersio JF. Diabetes mellitus as a poor mobilizer condition. *Blood Rev* [Internet]. 2018 Nov 8;32(3):184–91. Available from: http://www.ncbi.nlm.nih.gov/pubmed/29132746.

[132] Albiero M, Menegazzo L, Boscaro E, Agostini C, Avogaro A, Fadini GPP. Defective recruitment, survival and proliferation of bone marrow-derived progenitor cells at sites of delayed diabetic wound healing in mice. *Diabetologia* [Internet]. 2011 Apr;54(4):945–53. Available from: http://www.ncbi.nlm.nih.gov/pubmed/21165593.

[133] Bolli R, Ghafghazi S. Stem cells: Cell therapy for cardiac repair: what is needed to move forward? *Nat Rev Cardiol* [Internet]. 2017;14(5):257–8. Available from: http://dx.doi.org/10.1038/nrcardio.2017.38.

[134] Yao L, Heuser-Baker J, Herlea-Pana O, Iida R, Wang Q, Zou M, et al. Bone Marrow Endothelial Progenitors Augment Atherosclerotic Plaque Regression in a Mouse Model of Plasma Lipid Lowering. *Stem Cells* [Internet]. 2012 Dec 27;30(12):2720–31. Available from: https://onlinelibrary.wiley.com/doi/10.1002/stem.1256.

[135] Kashiwazaki D, Koh M, Uchino H, Akioka N, Kuwayama N, Noguchi K, et al. Hypoxia accelerates intraplaque neovascularization derived from endothelial progenitor cells in carotid stenosis. *J Neurosurg* [Internet]. 2018;131(3):884–91. Available from: http://www.ncbi.nlm.nih.gov/pubmed/30485214.

[136] Michel JB, Virmani R, Arbustini E, Pasterkamp G. Intraplaque haemorrhages as the trigger of plaque vulnerability. *Eur Heart J.* 2011;32(16):1977–85.

[137] Hagensen MK, Raarup MK, Mortensen MB, Thim T, Nyengaard JR, Falk E, et al. Circulating endothelial progenitor cells do not contribute to regeneration of endothelium after murine arterial injury. *Cardiovasc Res.* 2012;93(2):223–31.

[138] Rigato M, Bittante C, Albiero M, Avogaro A, Fadini GPGP. Circulating progenitor cell count predicts microvascular outcomes in type 2 diabetic patients. *J Clin Endocrinol Metab* [Internet]. 2015;100(7):2666–72. Available from: https://academic.oup.com/jcem/article-lookup/doi/10.1210/jc.2015-1687.

[139] Asnaghi V, Lattanzio R, Mazzolari G, Pastore MR, Ramoni A, Maestroni A, et al. Increased clonogenic potential of circulating endothelial progenitor cells in patients with type 1 diabetes and proliferative retinopathy [2]. *Diabetologia* [Internet]. 2006;49(5):1109–11. Available from: http://link.springer.com/10.1007/s00125-006-0180-0.

[140] Liu X, Li Y, Liu Y, Luo Y, Wang D, Annex BH, et al. Endothelial progenitor cells (EPCs) mobilized and activated by neurotrophic factors may contribute to pathologic neovascularization in diabetic retinopathy. *Am J Pathol* [Internet]. 2010;176(1):504–15. Available from: http://dx.doi.org/10.2353/ajpath.2010.081152.

[141] Lee IG, Chae SL, Kim JC. Involvement of circulating endothelial progenitor cells and vasculogenic factors in the pathogenesis of diabetic retinopathy. *Eye* (Lond) [Internet]. 2006 May;20(5):546–52. Available from: http://www.ncbi.nlm.nih.gov/pubmed/15905870.

[142] Mathur A, Fernandez-Aviles F, Bartunek J, Belmans A, Crea F, Dowlut S, et al. The effect of intracoronary infusion of bone marrow-derivedmononuclear cells on all-cause mortality in acutemyocardial infarction: The BAMI trial. *Eur Heart J.* 2020;41(38):3702–10.

[143] Bak RO, Dever DP, Porteus MH. CRISPR/Cas9 genome editing in human hematopoietic stem cells. *Nat Protoc* [Internet]. 2018;13(2):358–76. Available from: http://www.ncbi.nlm.nih.gov/pubmed/29370156.

[144] Krohn-Grimberghe M, Mitchell MJ, Schloss MJ, Khan OF, Courties G, Guimaraes PPGG, et al. Nanoparticle-encapsulated siRNAs for gene silencing in the haematopoietic stem-cell niche. *Nat Biomed Eng* [Internet]. 2020;4(11):1076–89. Available from: http://dx.doi.org/10.1038/s41551-020-00623-7.

[145] Fadini GP, Pucci L, Vanacore R, Baesso I, Penno G, Balbarini A, et al. Glucose tolerance is negatively associated with circulating progenitor cell levels. *Diabetologia.* 2007;50(10):2156–63.

[146] Egan CG, Lavery R, Caporali F, Fondelli C, Laghi-Pasini F, Dotta F, et al. Generalised reduction of putative endothelial progenitors and CXCR4-positive peripheral blood cells in type 2 diabetes. *Diabetologia* [Internet]. 2008 Jul;51(7):1296–305. Available from: http://www.ncbi.nlm.nih.gov/pubmed/18286257.

[147] Pirro M, Schillaci G, Paltriccia R, Bagaglia F, Menecali C, Mannarino MR, et al. Increased ratio of CD31+/CD42- microparticles to endothelial progenitors as a novel marker of atherosclerosis in hypercholesterolemia. *Arterioscler Thromb Vasc Biol* [Internet]. 2006 Nov;26(11):2530–5. Available from: http://www.ncbi.nlm.nih.gov/pubmed/16946129.

Section IV: Clinical EPC Transplantation Trials

Chapter 5

Endothelial Progenitor Cell Therapy in Heart Disease – Pitfalls in Clinical Translation, Impact of Stem Cell Senescence, and Personalized Medicine by AI-Application

Gustav Steinhoff[1,*] **and Markus Wolfien**[2,†]
[1]Cardiac Surgery, Department Life,
Light and Matter, University Rostock, Rostock, Germany
[2]University Rostock, Institute of Computer Science,
Department of Systems Biology and Bioinformatics,
Rostock, Germany

Abstract

Endothelial precursor cell (EPC) based regenerative therapies have raised highest expectation after successful preclinical evidence of therapeutic effectiveness. However, the clinical translation in heart failure was not yet successful in randomized controlled trials. Research analysis of clinical trials revealed genetic and epigenetic damage to stem and progenitor cells in acquired adult disease mechanisms affecting stem cell function. EPC were modified by somatic mutations and epigenetic DNA-pathology leading to aberrant clonal disease mechanisms. To identify the responsible pathways in clinical disease a close interdisciplinary

* Corresponding Author's Email: gustav.steinhoff@uni-rostock.de.
† Corresponding Author's Email: markus.wolfien@uni-rostock.de.

In: Endothelial Progenitor Cells in Health and Disease
Editors: Amankeldi A. Salybekov, Shuzo Kobayashi and Takayuki Asahara
ISBN: 978-1-68507-794-5

approach is needed crossing medical and nonmedical disciplines. To identify novel disease diagnostics in stem/immune cells, there is a need to improve individualized diagnostics of underlying disease of stem cells. Precision medicine and artificial intelligence-based analysis can be used to unravel personalized diagnostic monitoring of molecular patho-mechanisms of EPC.

Keywords: EPC transplantation, clinical trials, stem cell therapy for cardiovascular diseases

Introduction

The discovery of the role of bone marrow derived circulating endothelial progenitor cells (EPC) in vascular regeneration more than two decades ago prompted intensive clinical research to use EPC to recover degenerated tissues in cardiovascular disease [1]. Since then, stem-cell-based regenerative therapies have raised highest expectation after successful preclinical evidence of therapeutic effectiveness. However, the clinical introduction has faced an unexpected failure in successful clinical translation [2]. Despite abundant evidence of induction of myocardial regeneration by intravascular and intramyocardial progenitor cell therapies using EPC, HSC, MSC, G-CSF, or erythropoietin, successful clinical evidence by level of significance in randomized controlled trials (RCT) has not been met [2, 3]. The suspected reason may be found in the principal genetic and epigenetic damage to stem and progenitor cells in acquired adult disease mechanisms [4]. A major difference of adult acquired cardiovascular disease to juvenile patients is accumulating DNA damage due to cell senescence by somatic mutations. This may be relevant to clinical translation by the lack of an equivalent disease status in preclinical animal models [2]. Immune progenitor cells, EPC, and MSC are prone to be modified by somatic mutations and epigenetic DNA-pathology leading to aberrant clonal disease mechanisms and progression upon mutagenic expansion [2]. To identify responsible pathways in clinical disease by altered genotype/phenotype patterns interfering with regenerative mechanisms, a close interdisciplinary approach is needed crossing medical and nonmedical disciplines. To identify novel disease diagnostics in stem/immune cells, there is a need to improve individualized diagnostics of underlying disease mechanisms using new technologies of artificial intelligence in systems medicine or deep learning methods. Stem cell senescence diagnostics in cardiovascular disease are needed to identify the impact of immune reaction and cardiac regeneration. Precision T-cell targeted and (stem) cell therapies modified by mRNA can be designed on the basis of personalized diagnostic monitoring of molecular pathomechanisms.

Vascular Regeneration and Angiogenesis Are Affected by Circulating EPC Pool

Circulating EPC represent a small population in adult peripheral blood comprising early committed cells at various maturation stages, with only little amounts of hematopoietic stem cells (HSC), endothelial progenitor cells (EPC) and mesenchymal stromal cells (MSC). Evidence has been generated more than 20 years ago that bone marrow-derived endothelial progenitor cells (EPCs) can be upregulated in the circulation to take part in postnatal angiogenesis and neovascularization [5-7]. Human EPCs co-express surface markers of both hematopoietic stem cells (CD34, CD117, and CD133 membrane expression) and endothelial cells (VEGF-R2 / KDR) [8]. EPCs differentiate into endothelial phenotype in culture and promote in vivo neovascularization and collateral formation in diabetic mice [9, 10].

In patients, peripheral blood circulating EPCs are reduced in coronary artery disease (CAD), endothelial dysfunction, smoking, hypercholesterolemia, and renal failure [11-16]. Reduced coronary collateral development is associated with reduced numbers of circulating EPCs [11, 12]. It is conceivable that depletion of circulating EPCs may contribute to both reduced angiogenesis and endothelial dysfunction, as an early event in the atherosclerotic process. In this context, circulating EPC reduction and dysfunction have been reported in both type 1 and type 2 diabetic patients [18-20]. Reduced EPC are thought to negatively affect postinfarction myocardial recovery [21].

Based on this theory initial clinical trials attempted the augmentation of circulating EPC by intracoronary autotransfusion of autologous bone marrow (BM) derived mononuclear cells (MNC) to counteract postinfarction myocardial degeneration [21]. In the first non-randomized controlled clinical trials the application of BM-MNCs in patients with acute myocardial infarction (MI) improved local contractility and perfusion, reduced left ventricular end-systolic volume (LVESV), and decreased infarction site compared with the standard therapy group [22]. The authors postulated that therapeutic effects were associated with myocardial regeneration and neovascularization. Since then, large numbers of clinical trials investigated the potential of BM-derived

MNCs for the treatment of ischemic and non-ischemic heart diseases [2]. However, therapeutic benefits have continued to remain controversial. In fact, several randomized, controlled studies demonstrated a significantly improved cardiac function after intravenous or intracoronary BM-derived MNC transplantation [23-25], while others could not prove cell-based benefits [26, 27]. This heterogenicity is also revealed by meta-analyses reporting an overall mild improvement of the global heart performance below 5% left ventricular ejection fraction (LVEF) and reduction of adverse cardiac remodeling [28], but also failed to detect therapeutic effects of BM-derived MNC on left ventricular function after acute myocardial infarction [29]. From research analysis in these trials patient heterogenicity in bone marrow function was identified as a potential cause of therapeutic inefficacy as compared to preclinical animal models lacking a design of stem cell failure [2, 29, 30].

Stem cell mobilization by systemic drug administration of granulocyte-colony stimulating factor (G-CSF) has experienced a similar outcome in clinical trials to stimulate the mobilization of stem and progenitor cells released from bone marrow [31-34]. Meta-analyses demonstrated that the G-CSF as a stand-alone therapy has no beneficial effects on myocardial regeneration [35, 36]. Late follow-up after 10 years, however, revealed signs of longstanding effects in myocardial remodeling [37]. The intramyocardial and intracoronary transplantation of G-CSF mobilized HSCs/EPCs also led to controversial results [38]. Nevertheless, feasibility and safety of intravascular BM-derived progenitor cell transfusion and pharmacological mobilization has been demonstrated in all of the Phase I and II clinical trials. Efficacy on disease outcomes has not been proven in pivotal phase III trials [2].

Observing a paradox of preclinical and clinical results leads to suspect differences in underlying disease mechanism. This open question was addressed in intensified clinical research programs on the mechanism of action of angiogenetic or immune response modulation by the German-Japanese PERFECT trial analysis [3], and the US - Cardiovascular Cell Therapy Research Network (CCTRN) [27].

Targeting EPC to Hypoperfused Ischemic Tissue: Intramyocardial Application

The first-in-man phase I trial for intramyocardial transplantation of purified $CD133^+$ BMSCs performed in Rostock in June 2001 revealed promising results of postinfarction induction of cardiac regeneration more than 10%

increase in LVEF [1]. The non-placebo randomized controlled phase IIa trial confirmed the finding of a significant LVEF increase in BMSC treated patients vs. coronary artery bypass graft (CABG) controls [39]. In a phase IIb placebo-controlled trial the BMSC induced improvement in heart function was not significantly different from placebo controls [40]. This was confirmed by the randomized double blinded placebo controlled multicenter phase III trial – PERFECT [3]. However, the overall increase in LVEF was 8,8% and a significant improvement in the heart function (LVEF > 5%) was observed in 60% of placebo, as well as stem cell treated patients [3]. Increase in LVEF was not different in the stem cell and placebo CABG treatment groups. In the PERFECT trial, 40% of patients were 'non-responders' to induction of cardiac regeneration irrespective their treatment with placebo or $CD133^{+}$ BMSCs. Induction of circulating EPCs, as well as angiogenesis and heart function improvement, was significantly reduced in non-responders [3]. Cardiac function improvement by purified intramyocardial BMSCs was effective only in patients with angiogenesis response by increase of circulating EPCs [3].

Biomarkers for EPC Angiogenesis Response in the PERFECT Trial

The PERFECT phase III trial included a study design with blood harvesting and storage before and at different intervals after CABG with or without EPC/HSC application [2]. In addition to FACS analyses of circulating EPC, the dynamics of more than 30 angiogenesis factors and cytokines were obtained at defined time intervals. Treatment responders were defined as having a ΔLVEF at 6 months versus baseline higher than 5%. Responder and non-responder but not $CD133^{+}$ stem cell and control groups differed in angiogenesis factors before operation. It was shown that non-responders display basically elevated angiogenesis stimulating factors as VEGF and EPO, as well as pro-inflammatory factor IP-10 and decreased level of IGFBP-3 accompanied by reduced amount and decreased induction of EPCs in PB. A low baseline level of VEGF in the responder group doubled in 10 days after CABG procedure [3]. The non-responders in the PERFECT trial show typically lowered $CD133^{+}/CD34^{+}/CD117^{+}$ EPC and reduced thrombocytes in peripheral blood (PB) combined to elevated angiogenesis stimulating factors, such as VEGF and EPO in the PB [3]. In contrast, responders display basically elevated EPCs and thrombocytes also in the absence of angiogenesis stimulating factors. The underlying mechanism for a lack of response to induction of cardiac regeneration may be a failure of vascular repair by reduced circulating EPCs. This mechanism relies on underlying disease in diabetic and atherosclerotic patients affecting EPC function and circulating levels [10-17]. Recent clinical findings on the association of BM failure and cardiovascular disease are setting the spotlight on BMSC function as the main disease pathomechanism. Altered BM subpopulations have been associated with response to stem cell therapy in CCTRN trial analysis [27]. Jaiswal et al. have found the association of BM-derived EPCs or altered clonal hematopoiesis and atherosclerotic cardiovascular disease [41, 42].

In the randomized PERFECT intramyocardial stem cell trial artificial intelligence (AI) methods including machine learning (ML) were used for analysis of preoperative predictive features for postoperative LVEF recovery. A preoperative signature of circulating BM-HSC/EPC and angiogenesis parameters in peripheral blood was significantly correlated to postoperative LVEF recovery [4]. Using RNA sequencing analysis in PB, a corresponding signature was identified for a decreased (NR) or enhanced (R) bone marrow stem cell response upon ischemic/inflammatory response to CABG. Gene expression patterns were found characteristic for a RvsNR preoperative steady state. These comprised pathways for proliferation control (*EGFR*, *PDFR*, *TCR*, *c-KIT*), inflammation (*IL2*, *IFN1*), and platelet activating factor synthesis (*LPCAT2*). Identified hub genes related to LVEF recovery and BM-HSC/EPC response were mainly genes coding for signaling, adaptor, and transcription regulation proteins [4].

Given the complexity of stem cell response to ischemic or inflammatory stimuli as induced by CABG-surgery, access to circuit pattern recognition in patients can only be found by unbiased ML methods. Learning from failed reductionistic attempts to define single control factors of stem cell reactivity, we propose this unbiased approach. Independent unbiased ML-based feature selection of RvsNR discriminating the most important factors gives evidence for a gene circuit effecting myocardial repair by modified expression of signaling and adaptor protein gene transcription [4]. The association of genes, such as *PLCG1*, *LPCAT2*, *AP1B1*, *AFAP1*, *GRB2*, *KLF8*, *MARK3*, with circulating $CD133^{+}/CD34^{+}$ cells, and serum proteins EPO/VEGF, were initially identified using ML and sequentially validated experimentally in mice models, as well as in an additional patient cohort. Further clustering analysis of the overall patient cohort revealed subgroups representing the complexity of gene expression, coexpression, and mutational variants [4]. Their functional interplay has to be studied in additional experimental models as exemplarily for the Src adaptor protein SH2B3/LNK that regulates crosstalk between integrin and cytokine signaling pathways in BM-HSC/megakaryocyte proliferation [4].

In the PERFECT trial genomic analysis multiple somatic mutations involving stem cell functional genes as *NOTCH2*, *PROM1/CD133*, *MTOR*, as well as the *SH2B3* gene were found in PB. In this context, mutations of *SH2B3/LNK* were present in all patients with a majority of responders expressing the exon variant RS3184504 that is associated to coronary artery disease and increased thrombocyte count. Human *SH2B3* gene expression was not linked to thrombocyte count and circulating $CD133^{+}/CD34^{+}$ BM-HSC, whereas correlation was found to LVEF response [4]. It is conceivable, that not reduced gene expression, but mutant related altered SH2B3/LNK protein signaling function impairs control of stem cell proliferation. Therefore, we compared gene expression patterns in a mouse model of CRISPR-Cas9-mediated SH2B3 knockout with human R/NR.

Similar to SH2B3/LNK in humans, LNK in the mouse model is an adaptor protein that negatively regulates multiple essential signals, including the SCF/c-KIT system, in stem/progenitor cells. In SH2B3/LNK deficient animals accelerated hindlimb ischemia recovery and bone fracture healing [42] is mainly achieved by restoring local blood perfusion with increased angiogenesis and osteogenesis, respectively. Following the series of SH2B3/LNK-related clinical observations in R/NR, we successfully demon-strated for the first-time clonal dominance in hematopoiesis, lymphopoiesis, and myelopoiesis by reduced SH2B3/LNK signaling. To test the hypothesis of a clonal network switch found in silico, we subsequently performed a competitive syngeneic bone marrow transplantation model in mice transplanted with unmodified and SH2B3/LNK knockout HSC. SH2B3/LNK knockout HSC clones displayed significant overgrowth of myeloid and immune cells in bone marrow, peripheral blood, and tissue at day 160 after BMT. Moreover, the gene expression profile of peripheral blood was similar to the human R/NR signature [4].

Furthermore, in ischemic myocardium using a $SH2B3/LNK^{-/-}$ mouse MI model, SH2B3/LNK deficiency increased the number of HSC/KSL stem/progenitor cells (including EPCs) in BM and stem/progenitor cells in myocardium [3]: Angiogenic growth factor, survival factor, and stem/progenitor chemokine mRNA expressions were up-regulated in SH2B3/LNK deficient BM/PB HSC stem/progenitor cells [4]. Significant mobilization of BM/PB stem/progenitor cells occurred following myocardial ischemia in SH2B3/LNK-negative mice and myocardial ischemic damage was reduced with increased angiogenesis to recruit BM-derived EPCs [4].

Clonal Dysregulation and Prediction of Response

Transcriptome data in the PERFECT trial revealed clonal HSC dysregulation prior to treatment. This was associated with specific disease phenotypes as reduced angiogenesis and sustained myocardial ischemia. HSC genotype was associated with cardiac recovery outcome in PERFECT trial coronary artery disease patients. Not specifically Clonal Hematopoiesis of Indeterminate Potential CHIP-gene mutations, but random mutations affecting distinct regulatory angiogenesis and HSC proliferation pathway gene mutations were observed [4]. These observations underline the hypothesis of coronary artery disease (CAD) as a phenotype of hematological stem cell disease and acquired senescence by somatic mutations in the tissue repair gene circuit [41, 42].

Based on these findings the approach to treat cardiovascular disease with stem cells has to be changed. It is noteworthy that the pathology of stem cells in the hematopoietic, immune, and vascular system forms the target of treatment of disease mechanism [2]. Moreover, only stem cells without pathological mutations in cell function can be considered safe tools for cell therapy purpose to repair tissue degeneration. For treatment thorough genetic analysis of underlying pathomechanism is mandatory f.i. to identify clonal overgrowth as well to classify altered proliferation, migration, or other cell functions. Switch genes of stem cell function as the SH2B3/LNK could be one interesting candidate for therapeutical intervention in proliferation and inflammation control [2].

Patient Selection and Individualized Therapy

Although the obtained data from the PERFECT trial with respect to AI-guided prediction of tissue regeneration response on basis of combined genotype/phenotype analysis are preliminary, the findings open a new pathway of diagnostic approaches to cardiovascular disease in peripheral blood [4]. Ongoing trials as the CardiAMP Heart Failure Trial to predict treatment response from colony forming capacity of bone marrow stem cells may deepen the diagnostic approach to bone marrow stem cell dysfunction [43]. Next phase studies are needed to build up a pathomechanism diagnosis classification based on genotype/phenotype analyses. It is obvious that AI-assisted diagnosis of stem cell based cardiac regeneration capacity in tissue ischemia, infection or vascular repair can be applied for differential diagnosis in heart disease [4].

Improved Therapeutic Concepts in the 21st Century with AI in EPC Therapy?

We now elaborate possible perspectives and drawbacks for clinicians and patients throughout this section to give rise to the question, if Artificial Intelligence (AI) is only overblown and hyped or a gatekeeper to cheaper and better medicine for EPC related therapeutic interventions. Since the first AI diagnostic system for MRI heart interpretation (Arterys, [44]) was approved from the FDA in 2017 many more followed with accelerating numbers (in total two in 2017, twelve in 2018 [45], 24 in 2019, and 51 in 2020) (https://aicentral.acrdsi.org/. Accessed at 20th October 2021) that might already suggest the increasing impact of AI in the upcoming future of healthcare in general (Figure 1).

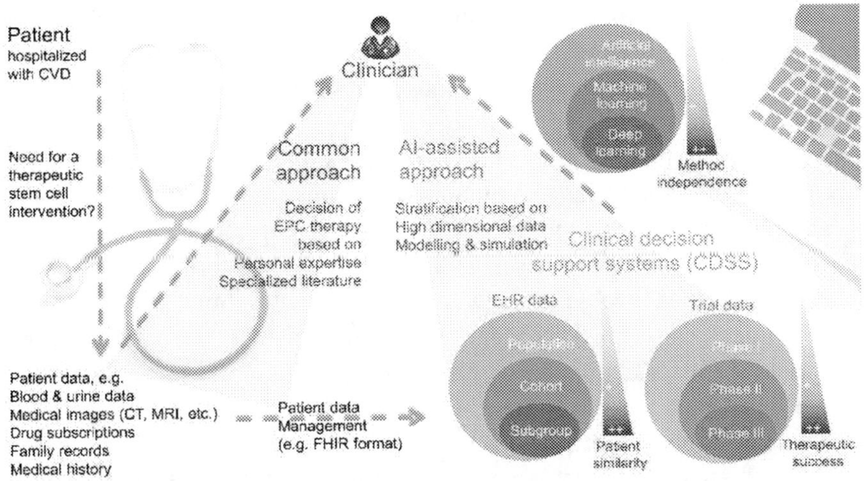

Figure 1. Comparison of common and AI-assisted EPC therapy decision making by clinicians. The common approach still remains but will be enhanced via novel technologies that support clinicians to overview and understand complex electronic health records (EHR), clinical trial data, and also currently available standard medical data in the Fast Healthcare Interoperable Resources (FHIR) format.

Although AI applications in medicine have a huge success, they still face a couple of hurdles and limitations. Also in EPC research, the evolution of digitalization in hospitals and the Good Clinical Practice (GCP) standards (i.e. Fast Healthcare Interoperable Resources, FHIR) led to a steadily increasing amount of good quality, structured, and machine interpretable data (i.e. electronic health record - EHR data). However, this data is currently only locally available at the specific hospital. Without universal data standards and common national or international compatible EHR formats the transferability between hospitals or even countries will remain a challenging, if not impossible to achieving, task. Such standards would lead to an absolutely needed increased sample size and would result in better and more robust AI models because the variety of patient data, including aforementioned mutations, would increase, which would generate in fact stronger predictions. Such AI systems and, likewise, Clinical Decision Support Systems (CDSS) would improve themselves with these newly obtained data [46]. Therefore, a globally established set of standards for EPC data management, structure, and privacy in addition to the technical infrastructure to maintain large amounts of data is inevitable, especially in the specific field of EPC research, to unravel the full potential of AI approaches on a larger scale (Figure 1).

AI models are less and less black boxes that lack full interpretability, which formerly was one reason for patients and clinicians to have a skeptical attitude towards this technology because it is comprehensible to mistrust unfamiliar interfaces and a hesitancy to give a machine or algorithm the responsibility of making life-critical decisions [47, 48]. For this reason, current research is focusing on supportive systems rather than systems that autonomously make decisions such as self-driving cars. In medicine, it is the human plus the machine rather versus the machine. Therefore, a CDSS should be seen as an extended tool for patient diagnostics that a clinician familiar with EPC treatment can utilize to judge on an individual therapeutic decision. Nevertheless, the former black box problem led to ongoing work on improved interpreting AI models, such as LIME [49], IBM's Trusted AI project [50], and Google's What-if project [51]. Ribeiro et al. [49] demonstrated that explanations are useful for a variety of models in trust-related tasks in the text and image domains with both expert and non-expert users: deciding between models, assessing trust, improving untrustworthy models, and getting insights into predictions. There are already numerous concepts with attribution to open the AI black-box mechanisms to be ultimately available for each clinician and patient to justify the AI model selection and the data elements that influenced their predictions and final decision to apply an EPC therapy [52, 53]. However, it is still very distinct interpreting a model on a technical level and likewise interpreting its decision about the underlying biology, but it is an appropriate start to find explanations and important features in AI model predictions [54]. Another important aspect to take into consideration is the combination of AI approaches and traditional mechanistic models (in vivo and in vitro) that are used to identify also the origin of a certain disease and not only predict the disease outcome because for reliable decisions it is necessary to comprehensively investigate its causes, as it was already demonstrated for SH2B3 in the EPC domain [55].

Several works are trying to raise awareness not only about choosing an appropriate metric to validate the models, but also to validate the models in a real-world clinical setting [45, 56]. Thus, the quality of a CDSS should not only be grounded in the performance metrics, but rather should be subjected to proof the clinically important improvements in relevant outcomes compared with usual standard care, along with the satisfaction of patients and clinicians, which is also a large opportunity for the EPC domain because tailormade treatments will be the key for an accurate and responsive therapeutic success.

Conclusion

AI will not be a panacea and if used improperly these systems can replicate or augment bad practices rather than improve clinical decisions [57]. Each AI application that is being potentially used, especially in the EPC domain in clinical use, has to be investigated and thoroughly questioned to be able to reveal its huge potential in patient treatment, in which individual, complex, and non-linear data need to be integrated within a yet a simple classification task [58].

If and only if this is being assured that both clinicians and patients will derive the trust needed to rely on this novel AI supported decisions, which maybe even more change the patient-clinician relationship than ten years ago evoked by Google's search engine. Patients and citizens at all have to be involved into these new technical developments to illustrate the benefits they can obtain [59]. Citizen Science projects would be an opportunity to introduce these great potentials of EPC use to a broader community of people, such as various other examples already demonstrated [60].

It will be inevitable for healthcare professionals and patients in the field of EPC and beyond to become familiar with AI technologies in the coming years to ensure that medical decisions in general or supported via CDSS and medical traffic-light-systems are used appropriately and the decisions made are comprehensible and as accurate as possible.

References

[1] Stamm C, Westphal B, Kleine H-D, Petzsch M, Kittner C, Klinge H, et al. Autologous bone-marrow stem-cell transplantation for myocardial regeneration. *Lancet.* 2003;361(9351):45–6.

[2] Steinhoff G, Nesteruk J, Wolfien M, Große J, Ruch U, Vasudevan P, et al. Stem cells and heart disease—Brake or accelerator? *Adv. Drug Deliv Rev.* 2017;120 (2239–2242):2–24.

[3] Steinhoff G, Nesteruk J, Wolfien M, Kundt G, Börgermann J, David R, et al. Cardiac function improvement and bone marrow response: Outcome analysis of the randomized PERFECT phase III clinical trial of intramyocardial CD133(+) application after myocardial infarction. *EBioMedicine.* 2017;22:208–224.

[4] Wolfien M, Klatt D, Salybekov AA, Ii M, Komatsu-Horii M, Gaebel R, et al. Hematopoietic stem-cell senescence and myocardial repair—Coronary artery disease genotype/phenotype analysis of post-MI myocardial regeneration response induced by CABG/CD133+ bone marrow hematopoietic stem cell treatment in RCT PERFECT Phase 3. *EBioMedicine.* 2020;57, 102862:102862.

[5] Asahara T, Murohara T, Sullivan A, Silver M, van der Zee R, Li T, et al. Isolation of putative progenitor endothelial cells for angiogenesis. *Science.* 1997;275(5302): 964–6.

[6] Asahara T, Masuda H, Takahashi T, Kalka C, Pastore C, Silver M, et al. Bone marrow origin of endothelial progenitor cells responsible for postnatal vasculogenesis in physiological and pathological neovascularization. *Circ Res.* 1999;85 (3):221–8.

[7] Hristov M. Endothelial progenitor cells isolation and characterization. *Trends Cardiovasc Med.* 2003;13(5):201–6.

[8] Salven P, Mustjoki S, Alitalo R, Alitalo K, Rafii S. VEGFR-3 and CD133 identify a population of CD34+ lymphatic/vascular endothelial precursor cells. *Blood.* 2003;101(1):168–72.

[9] Schatteman GC, Hanlon HD, Jiao C, Dodds SG, Christy BA. Blood-derived angioblasts accelerate blood-flow restoration in diabetic mice. *J Clin Invest.* 2000;106(4):571–8.

[10] Abacı A, Oğuzhan A, Kahraman S, Eryol NK, Ünal S, Arınç H, et al. Effect of diabetes mellitus on formation of coronary collateral vessels. *Circulation.* 1999; 99(17):2239–42.

[11] Vasa M, Fichtlscherer S, Aicher A, Adler K, Urbich C, Martin H, et al. Number and migratory activity of circulating endothelial progenitor cells inversely correlate with risk factors for coronary artery disease. *Circ Res* [Internet]. 2001;89(1). Available from: http://dx.doi.org/10.1161/hh1301.093953.

[12] Hill JM, Zalos G, Halcox JPJ, Schenke WH, Waclawiw MA, Quyyumi AA, et al. Circulating endothelial progenitor cells, vascular function, and cardiovascular risk. *N Engl J Med.* 2003;348(7):593–600.

[13] Chen J, Zhang F, Tao Q, Wang X, Zhu J. Number and activity of endothelial progenitor cells from peripheral blood in patients with hypercholesterolemia. *Clin Sci* (Lond. 2004;107 273–280.

[14] Kondo T, Hayashi M, Takeshita K, Numaguchi Y, Kobayashi K, Iino S, et al. Smoking cessation rapidly increases circulating progenitor cells in peripheral blood in chronic smokers. *Arterioscler Thromb Vasc Biol.* 2004;24(8):1442–7.

[15] Choi J-H, Kim KL, Huh W, Kim B, Byun J, Suh W, et al. Decreased number and impaired angiogenic function of endothelial progenitor cells in patients with chronic renal failure. *Arterioscler Thromb Vasc Biol.* 2004;24(7):1246–52.

[16] Lambiase PD, Edwards RJ, Anthopoulos P, Rahman S, Meng YG, Bucknall CA, et al. Circulating humoral factors and endothelial progenitor cells in patients with differing coronary collateral support. *Circulation.* 2004;109(24):2986–92.

[17] Tepper OM, Galiano RD, Capla JM, Kalka C, Gagne PJ, Jacobowitz GR, et al. Human endothelial progenitor cells from type II diabetics exhibit impaired proliferation, adhesion, and incorporation into vascular structures. *Circulation.* 2002;106(22):2781–6.

[18] Waltenberger J. Impaired collateral vessels development in diabetes: potential cellular mechanisms and therapeutic implications. *Cardiovasc Res.* 2001;49:554–560.

[19] Tamarat R, Silvestre J-S, Le Ricousse-Roussanne S, Barateau V, Lecomte-Raclet L, Clergue M, et al. Impairment in ischemia-induced neovascularization in diabetes: bone marrow mononuclear cell dysfunction and therapeutic potential of placenta growth factor treatment. *Am J Pathol.* 2004;164(2):457–66.

[20] Loomans CJM, de Koning EJP, Staal FJT, Rookmaaker MB, Verseyden C, de Boer HC, et al. Endothelial progenitor cell dysfunction: a novel concept in the pathogenesis of vascular complications of type 1 diabetes. *Diabetes.* 2004;53(1): 195–9.

[21] Shintani S, Murohara T, Ikeda H, Ueno T, Honma T, Katoh A, et al. Mobilization of endothelial progenitor cells in patients with acute myocardial infarction. *Circulation.* 2001;103(23):2776–9.

[22] Strauer BE, Brehm M, Zeus T, Gattermann N, Hernandez A, Sorg RV, et al. Intrakoronare, humane autologe Stammzelltransplantation zur Myokardregeneration nach Herzinfarkt [*Intracoronary, human autologous stem cell transplantation for myocardial regeneration after heart attack*]. *Dtsch Med Wochenschr.* 2001;126(34/35):932–8.

[23] Schächinger V, Erbs S, Elsässer A, Haberbosch W, Hambrecht R, Hölschermann H, et al. Intracoronary bone marrow-derived progenitor cells in acute myocardial infarction. *N Engl J Med.* 2006;355(12):1210–21.

[24] Wollert KC, Meyer GP, Lotz J, Ringes-Lichtenberg S, Lippolt P, Breidenbach C, et al. Intracoronary autologous bone-marrow cell transfer after myocardial infarction: the BOOST randomised controlled clinical trial. *Lancet.* 2004; 364 (9429):141–8.

[25] Huikuri HV, Kervinen K, Niemelä M, Ylitalo K, Säily M, Koistinen P, et al. Effects of intracoronary injection of mononuclear bone marrow cells on left ventricular function, arrhythmia risk profile, and restenosis after thrombolytic therapy of acute myocardial infarction. *Eur Heart J.* 2008;29(22):2723–32.

[26] Sürder D, Manka R, Lo Cicero V, Moccetti T, Rufibach K, Soncin S, et al. Intracoronary injection of bone marrow-derived mononuclear cells early or late

after acute myocardial infarction: effects on global left ventricular function. *Circulation.* 2013;127(19):1968–79.

[27] Traverse JH, Henry TD, Ellis SG, Pepine CJ, Willerson JT, Zhao DXM, et al. Effect of intracoronary delivery of autologous bone marrow mononuclear cells 2 to 3 weeks following acute myocardial infarction on left ventricular function: the LateTIME randomized trial: The LateTIME randomized trial. *JAMA.* 2011;306 (19):2110–9.

[28] Yang D, O'Brien CG, Ikeda G, Traverse JH, Taylor DA, Henry TD, et al. Meta-analysis of short- and long-term efficacy of mononuclear cell transplantation in patients with myocardial infarction. *Am Heart J.* 2020;220:155–75.

[29] Contreras A, For the Cardiovascular Cell Therapy Research Network (CCTRN), Orozco AF, Resende M, Schutt RC, Traverse JH, et al. Identification of cardiovascular risk factors associated with bone marrow cell subsets in patients with STEMI: a biorepository evaluation from the CCTRN TIME and LateTIME clinical trials. *Basic Res Cardiol* [Internet]. 2017;112(1). Available from: http://dx.doi.org/10.1007/s00395-016-0592-z.

[30] Tompkins BA, Balkan W, Winkler J, Gyöngyösi M, Goliasch G, Fernández-Avilés F, et al. Preclinical studies of stem cell therapy for heart disease. *Circ Res.* 2018;122(7):1006–20.

[31] Wang X, Chacon LI, Derakhshandeh R, Rodriguez HJ, Han DD, Kostyushev DS, et al. Impaired therapeutic efficacy of bone marrow cells from post-myocardial infarction patients in the TIME and LateTIME clinical trials. *PLoS One.* 2020; 15(8):e0237401.

[32] Sheridan WP, Begley CG, Juttner CA, Szer J, To LB, Maher D, et al. Effect of peripheral-blood progenitor cells mobilised by filgrastim (G-CSF) on platelet recovery after high-dose chemotherapy. *Lancet.* 1992;339(8794):640–4.

[33] Zohlnhöfer D, Dibra A, Koppara T, de Waha A, Ripa RS, Kastrup J, et al. Stem cell mobilization by granulocyte colony-stimulating factor for myocardial recovery after acute myocardial infarction: a meta-analysis. *J Am Coll Cardiol.* 2008;51(15): 1429–37.

[34] Abdel-Latif A, Bolli R, Zuba-Surma EK, Tleyjeh IM, Hornung CA, Dawn B. Granulocyte colony-stimulating factor therapy for cardiac repair after acute myocardial infarction: a systematic review and meta-analysis of randomized controlled trials. *Am Heart J.* 2008;156(2):216-226.e9.

[35] Kang H-J, Kim H-S, Zhang S-Y, Park K-W, Cho H-J, Koo B-K, et al. Effects of intracoronary infusion of peripheral blood stem-cells mobilised with granulocyte-colony stimulating factor on left ventricular systolic function and restenosis after coronary stenting in myocardial infarction: the MAGIC cell randomised clinical trial. *Lancet.* 2004;363(9411):751–6.

[36] Kang H-J, Lee H-Y, Na S-H, Chang S-A, Park K-W, Kim H-K, et al. Differential effect of intracoronary infusion of mobilized peripheral blood stem cells by granulocyte colony-stimulating factor on left ventricular function and remodeling in patients with acute myocardial infarction versus old myocardial infarction: the MAGIC Cell-3-DES randomized, controlled trial: The MAGIC cell-3-DES randomized, controlled trial. *Circulation.* 2006;114(1 Suppl):I145-51.

[37] Moazzami K, Roohi A, Moazzami B. Granulocyte colony stimulating factor therapy for acute myocardial infarction. *Cochrane Database Syst Rev.* 2013;2021(5):CD-008844.

[38] Leone AM, D'Amario D, Cannata F, Graziani F, Borovac JA, Leone G, et al. The effects of granulocyte colony-stimulating factor in patients with a large anterior wall acute myocardial infarction to prevent left ventricular remodeling: A 10-year follow-up of the RIGENERA study. *J Clin Med.* 2020;9(4):1214.

[39] Stamm C, Kleine H-D, Choi Y-H, Dunkelmann S, Lauffs J-A, Lorenzen B, et al. Intramyocardial delivery of CD133+ bone marrow cells and coronary artery bypass grafting for chronic ischemic heart disease: Safety and efficacy studies. *J Thorac Cardiovasc Surg.* 2007;133(3):717-725.e5.

[40] Nasseri BA, Ebell W, Dandel M, Kukucka M, Gebker R, Doltra A, et al. Autologous CD133+ bone marrow cells and bypass grafting for regeneration of ischaemic myocardium: the Cardio133 trial. *Eur Heart J.* 2014;35(19):1263–74.

[41] Jaiswal S, Fontanillas P, Flannick J, Manning A, Grauman PV, Mar BG, et al. Age-related clonal hematopoiesis associated with adverse outcomes. *N Engl J Med.* 2014;371(26):2488–98.

[42] Jaiswal S, Natarajan P, Silver AJ, Gibson CJ, Bick AG, Shvartz E, et al. Clonal hematopoiesis and risk of atherosclerotic cardiovascular disease. *N Engl J Med.* 2017;377(2):111–21.

[43] Raval AN, Johnston PV, Duckers HJ, Cook TD, Traverse JH, Altman PA, et al. Point of care, bone marrow mononuclear cell therapy in ischemic heart failure patients personalized for cell potency: 12-month feasibility results from CardiAMP heart failure roll-in cohort. *Int J Cardiol.* 2021;326:131–8.

[44] Marr B. *First FDA Approval for Clinical Cloud-Based Deep Learning in Healthcare.* https://www.forbes.com/sites/bernardmarr/2017/01/20/first-fda-approval-for-clinical-cloud-based-deep-learning-in-healthcare/. 2017.

[45] Topol EJ. High-performance medicine: the convergence of human and artificial intelligence. *Nat Med.* 2019 Jan;25(1):44–56.

[46] Jiang F, Jiang Y, Zhi H, Dong Y, Li H, Ma S, et al. Artificial intelligence in healthcare: past, present and future. *Stroke Vasc Neurol.* 2017 Dec;2(4):230–43.

[47] Begoli E, Bhattacharya T, Kusnezov D. The need for uncertainty quantification in machine-assisted medical decision making. *Nat Mach Intell.* 2019 Jan;1(1):20–3.

[48] Rudin C. Stop explaining black box machine learning models for high stakes decisions and use interpretable models instead. *Nat Mach Intell.* 2019;1(5):206–15.

[49] Ribeiro MT, Singh S, Guestrin C. "Why should i trust you?" Explaining the predictions of any classifier. *KDD '16: Proceedings of the 22nd ACM SIGKDD International Conference on Knowledge Discovery and Data Mining*. 2016. https://arxiv.org/abs/1602.04938. 2016.

[50] IBM. *Trusted AI - Artificial Intelligence - IBM Research.* https://research.ibm.com/teams/trusted-ai. 2019.

[51] Google. *What-If Tool.* https://cloud.google.com/ai-platform/prediction/docs/using-what-if-tool. 2019.

[52] Koh PW, Liang P. Understanding black-box predictions via influence functions. *International Conference on Machine Learning*. 2017. https://arxiv.org/abs/1703.04730. 2017 Mar.

[53] Lei D, Chen X, Zhao J. Opening the black box of deep learning *arXiv Preprint arXiv:1805.08355.* https://arxiv.org/ abs/1805.08355. 2018.

[54] Avati A, Jung K, Harman S, Downing L, Ng A, Shah NH. Improving Palliative Care with Deep Learning. *BMC Med Inform Decis Mak.* 2017 Nov.

[55] Baker RE, Peña J-M, Jayamohan J, Jérusalem A. Mechanistic models versus machine learning, a fight worth fighting for the biological community? *Biol Lett.* 2018 May;14(5):20170660.

[56] Cabitza F, Rasoini R, Gensini GF. Unintended consequences of machine learning in medicine. *JAMA.* 2017 Aug;318(6):517.

[57] Gottesman O, Johansson F, Komorowski M, Faisal A, Sontag D, Doshi-Velez F, et al. Guidelines for reinforcement learning in healthcare. *Nat Med.* 2019 Jan;25(1): 16–8.

[58] Keane PA, Topol EJ. With an eye to AI and autonomous diagnosis. *Npj Digit Med.* 2018 Dec;1(1):40.

[59] Guerrini CJ, Contreras JL. Credit for and control of research outputs in genomic citizen science. *Annu Rev Genomics Hum Genetics.* https://doi.org/101146/annurev-genom-083117-021812. 2020 Sep 1; 21:465–89.

[60] Shell L. The future is here: Artificial Intelligence meets Citizen Science. *CitizenSci.* 2019.

Chapter 6

EPC in Peripheral Arterial Diseases

Yasuyuki Fujita and Atsuhiko Kawamoto*
Translational Research Center for Medical Innovation,
Foundation for Biomedical Research and Innovation at Kobe,
Kobe, Japan

Abstract

Chronic critical limb ischemia (CLI) represents an end-stage manifestation of peripheral arterial disease (PAD). CLI patients are at very high risk of amputation and cardiovascular complications, leading to severe morbidity and mortality. This chapter provides an overview of preclinical and clinical reports to demonstrate the usefulness and prospects of endothelial progenitor cell (EPC)-based therapies.

Keywords: arteriosclerosis obliterans (ASO), critical limb ischemia (CLI), peripheral arterial disease (PAD), thromboangiitis obliterans (TAO)

Introduction

Peripheral arterial disease (PAD), which is a circulation disorder caused by the stenosis or occlusion of arteries in the limbs, is estimated to affect more than 200 million individuals globally [1], ranging from asymptomatic to severe. The most common underlying disease is arteriosclerosis obliterans

* Corresponding Author's Email: kawamoto@fbri.org.

In: Endothelial Progenitor Cells in Health and Disease
Editors: Amankeldi A. Salybekov, Shuzo Kobayashi and Takayuki Asahara
ISBN: 978-1-68507-794-5

(ASO) caused mainly by atherosclerosis; other underlying diseases include thromboangiitis obliterans (TAO) (also known as Buerger's disease), vasculitis, and autoimmune diseases.

Chronic critical limb ischemia (CLI) is defined as advanced PAD, due to which patients experience pain at rest and have ulcers or gangrene on their lower limbs (Fontaine classification stage III or more severe, or Rutherford classification category 4 or more severe) that persists for two weeks or longer. CLI is the end stage of PAD, and generally has been observed to have a very poor prognosis, being comparable with those of some advanced malignancies. It has a mortality rate of 25%, a survival rate of 30% after major amputation, and a CLI persistence rate of 20% at 1 year after diagnosis of CLI. Furthermore, CLI patients have a 5-year survival rate of 40–50% [2]. The annual incidence of CLI is 500–1,000 per million in Europe and the United States. An estimated 250,000 amputations of lower limbs were performed annually because of CLI [1]. The global number of patients with PAD has increased by 23.5% between 2000 and 2010 [2], and there is concern that the number of PAD patients may increase rapidly in the future. The amputation of the lower limbs not only seriously deteriorates the patient's quality of life, but also causes major social and economic loss.

The currently recommended therapeutic interventions for CLI include pain control, risk factor management, treatment of ulcers or gangrene, and for suitable patients, revascularization by bypass surgery or endovascular repair [3]. However, revascularization is unsuitable for approximately 25–40% of CLI patients because they lack the vein grafts needed for the bypass surgery or have multiple extensive artery lesions or comorbidities [4, 1, 5]. The primary goal of the CLI treatment is to save the patient's life and limbs. Given that patients who are not suitable for revascularization or have refractory conditions have a very poor prognosis, it is socially and medically imperative to develop a treatment strategy for such 'no-option' CLI patients.

Nonclinical Studies

Kalka et al. obtained endothelial progenitor cells (EPCs) by culturing peripheral blood mononuclear cells (PBMNCs) from healthy subjects, and transplanted EPCs into the nude mouse model of hindlimb ischemia. When the EPCs were intravenously injected after two days of hindlimb ischemia, accumulation of the transplanted cells at the site of ischemia was histologically confirmed, indicating that the EPCs contributed to neovascularization in collaboration with mouse-derived vascular endothelial cells. Cell transplantation significantly improved the capillary density observed histologically and blood perfusion in the ischemic limbs as measured by laser Doppler flowmetry. As a result, the limb salvage rate from necrosis due to severe ischemia was 59% in the EPC transplantation group, compared with only 7–8% in the control group [6]. Murohara et al. reported similar positive results after they transplanted the EPCs collected by culturing human umbilical cord blood into nude rats with hindlimb ischemia [7]. Losordo et al. also obtained favorable results after they collected and isolated CD34+ cells from the PBMNCs of healthy subjects who had received a subcutaneous injection of G-CSF and transplanted CD34+ cells into nude rats with hindlimb ischemia (unpublished data).

Nonclinical studies have also shown that EPC transplantation therapy is effective for treating other diseases, such as myocardial infarction [8, 9], cerebral infarction [10], and refractory fracture [11]. These results theoretically not only support EPC transplantation, but also support the transplantation of bone marrow derived mononuclear cells (BMMNCs, a cell group that includes hematopoietic and mesenchymal cells as well as EPCs). The EPCs transplanted into the animal model of ischemia were directly integrated into new blood vessels in the ischemic tissue by vasculogenesis to form the vascular endothelium. The transplanted EPCs were found to produce various cytokines and vascular growth factors involved in angiogenesis, such as vascular endothelial growth factor, hepatic growth factor, angiopoietin-1, stromal-cell-derived factor-1 alpha, insulin-like growth factor-1, and endothelial nitric oxide synthase [12, 13, 14], promoting the proliferation of the existing vascular endothelium and cellular migration, which is called 'the paracrine effect'. Moreover, EPCs have been shown to release not only angiogenesis-related proteins, but also ribonucleic acids (RNAs) and exosomes containing microRNA, which contribute to the paracrine effect via gene-control mechanisms [15, 16]. While the therapeutic usefulness of purified EPCs (CD34+ cells) isolated from BMMNCs or PBMNCs have been demonstrated, transplantation of BMMNCs or PBMNCs without purifying EPCs have been attempted in several nonclinical studies because of procedural ease.

However, several studies have highlighted the risks associated with transplanting mixed cell groups, including ossification by osteoblasts, chondrification by chondroblasts, and fibrosis by fibroblasts. A nonclinical study by Yoon et al. showed that myocardial calcification occurred with a high frequency when whole bone marrow cells were transplanted intramyocardially into the rat model of acute myocardial ischemia [17]. Kawamoto et al. have also demonstrated that the intramyocardial transplantation of high-dose PBMNCs into the rat model of acute myocardial ischemia led to intramyocardial hemorrhage with the infiltration of several inflammatory cells and a reduced improvement in neovascularization and cardiac function. In contrast, the transplantation of purified CD34+ cells alone was associated with an absence of adverse reactions, high levels of neovascularization, and sustained recovery of cardiac function [9]. The *in vitro* EPC colony-forming assay developed by Masuda et al. showed that EPC colonies are formed from CD34+ cells at a high frequency, whereas colonies could not be obtained from CD34− mononuclear cells even when using 100 times more cells, demonstrating a marked difference in the vascularization potential between the EPC and non-EPC fractions [18]. These fundamental research and nonclinical studies suggest that the transplantation of purified EPCs is superior to BMMNC or PBMNC transplantation in terms of low invasiveness, therapeutic effect, and safety.

Clinical Studies

Physiological Significance of EPCs

Some reports have shown that patients with diabetes mellitus and patients with multiple risk factors for arteriosclerosis have fewer EPCs circulating in their PB in comparison with healthy individuals and that EPCs in these patients have lower proliferative and migratory capacities [19, 20]. Notably, arteriosclerosis patients with fewer EPCs in circulation have several risk factors for poor cardiovascular prognoses and reduced vascular endothelial function [21]. Thus, EPCs have been shown to be one of the important intrinsic factors that determine the prognosis of patients with arteriosclerosis.

Cell Types, Methods of Administration, and Endpoints of Clinical Trials

Crude BMMNCs or PBMNCs, including EPCs as well as the EPC-enriched fraction purified from the crude MNCs have been preclinically applied for ischemic cardiovascular diseases, including PAD. The promising results from these experimental studies in rodents promoted the initiation of clinical pilot trials. The cell sources are mainly BM or granulocyte-colony stimulating factor (G-CSF) mobilized PB. Crude MNCs are usually separated by density gradient centrifugation or leukapheresis. Fractionated CD34+ cells are further purified from crude MNCs using an antibody-coated magnetic bead sorting technique. Intramuscular or intraarterial administration has been selected as the route of cell administration. The efficacy endpoints, including amputation-free survival (AFS), ulcer healing, Rutherford's category, Fontaine classification, ankle-brachial pressure index (ABI), toe-brachial pressure index (TBI), transcutaneous oxygen pressure ($TcPO_2$), rest pain scale, walking distance, and quality of life (QOL) have been used.

Bone Marrow Mononuclear Cells

In 2002, the first clinical trial of intramuscular implantation of BMMNCs was reported in patients with PAD [22]. BMMNC therapy resulted in the improvement of rest pain, ABI, $TcPO_2$, and pain-free walking distance at 24 weeks follow up compared with the baseline. Improvement of rest pain, ulcer size, and pain-free walking distance was maintained 2 years after the BMMNC therapy [23]. Subsequent studies have investigated the safety, efficacy, and feasibility of BMMNCs for the treatment of ischemic limbs, mainly in small case series.

Since 2010s, randomized controlled trials have been conducted and provided additional evidence. In the PROVASA (Intraarterial Progenitor Cell Transplantation of Bone Marrow Mononuclear Cells for Induction of Neovascularization in Patients with Peripheral Arterial Occlusive Disease) trial conducted in Germany [24], which was a multicenter, randomized, double-blind, placebo-controlled trial of BMMNC therapy, a total of 40 patients with CLI were enrolled, received either intraarterial administration of BMMNCs or placebo. At the end of 3 months, the placebo group were crossed over to active treatment (an initial administration of BMMNCs) and the active group received the second administration of BMMNCs. This study demonstrated a dose-dependent improvement in ulcer healing and significant reduction in the rest pain, despite no difference in the limb salvage rate, amputation-free survival, and the primary endpoint, which was an increase in the ABI between the groups (Table 1). Furthermore, in the patients with Rutherford's category 6 (extensive gangrene and impending amputation), the CLI at baseline did not respond to the administration of BM-MNCs. All the patients with Rutherford's category 6 at baseline underwent major amputation within 3 months after the treatment, presumably owing to rapid progression of the disease. The PROVASA investigators speculated that the choice of change in ABI as the primary endpoint was inappropriate because the change of ABI did not correlate with improvements in the clinically most relevant endpoints, including ulcer healing and rest pain reduction.

The discordance between the clinical endpoints and functional endpoints, such as ABI, TBI, or $TcPO_2$ was similarly reported in a gene therapy trial for therapeutic angiogenesis in CLI [25] and remains a cardinal issue in the design and execution of clinical trials in CLI. In the JUVENTAS (Rejuvenating Endothelial Progenitor Cells via Transcutaneous Intra-arterial Supplementation) randomized, double-blind, placebo-controlled clinical trial conducted in the Netherlands [26], 160 patients with severe (Rutherford's category 3–6), nonrevascularizable limb ischemia were randomly assigned to receive repetitive intraarterial infusion (3 times; 3-week interval) of BMMNCs or placebo. The primary endpoint of this clinical trial was major amputation through or above the ankle joint within 6 months after randomization. This clinical trial demonstrated no significant differences of major amputation at 6 months between the BMMNC and the placebo groups. The secondary outcomes, including QOL, rest pain, ABI, and $TcPO_2$ improved during follow-up in the BMMNC group; however, there were no significant differences of the improvements between the groups (Table 1). The investigator concluded that further study is warranted to evaluate whether a therapeutic strategy with selected cell populations or different modes of administration may provide further benefit in patients with advanced PAD. Although the initial non-placebo controlled and small studies demonstrated advantages of BMMNC therapy, the larger placebo-controlled trials showed fewer convincing results on hard endpoints, such as amputation, limb salvage, and AFS.

In Japan, on the other hand, the intramuscular transplantation of BMMNC for CLI was approved in 2003 as 'Highly Advanced Medical Technology', which was reorganized and renamed to 'Advanced Medical Care Program (AMCP) – type A' from 2006, due to the Act Partially Amending the Health Insurance Act, etc. (Act No. 83 of 2006) by the Ministry of Health, Labor, and Welfare. AMCP consists of two categories, type A and type B. AMCPs using pharmaceutically approved and minimally invasive new technologies are categorized as AMCP-type A, whereas AMCPs using unapproved medical products or those using approved but highly invasive new technologies are categorized into AMCP-type B. A total of 345 CLI patients (168 patients with ASO, 108 patients with TAO, and 69 patients with collagen disease-related vasculitis [CDV]) received intramuscular transplantation of BMMNCs. The retrospective observational study for these patients revealed that the 10-year AFS rates for patients with ASO, TAO, and CDV were 37.8%, 80.9%, and 61.2%, respectively [27]. The results show that the intramuscular transplantation of BMMNCs was expected to be most effective in CLI patients with TAO. In order to further verify the effect, a multicenter clinical trial for CLI patients with TAO has been started in 2018 as AMCP-type B.

G-CSF-Mobilized PBMNCs

G-CSF-mobilized PBMNC therapy has been also investigated in CLI. PBMNCs are usually mobilized using several doses of subcutaneous G-CSF and harvested by leukapheresis. The intramuscular injection of unfractionated, mobilized PBMNCs improved ABI, $TcPO_2$, and ulcer healing in small-sized, randomized, clinical trials [28, 29]. Horie et al. conducted a phase III IMPACT (Improvement of Peripheral Arterial Disease by Granulocyte Colony-Stimulating Factor-Mobilized Autologous Peripheral-Blood-Mononuclear Cell Transplantation) trial in patients with PAD caused by ASO or TAO in Japan [30]. The primary endpoint was progression-free survival (PFS) within one year after allocation. The progression was defined as worsening of Rutherford's category, an increase in the skin ulcer size, gangrene extension, a new ulcer or gangrene, or major amputation. This study enrolled a total of 107 PAD patients. At baseline, Fontaine Classification was stage II–III in 82 patients and stage IV in 21 patients, and 54 patients were on hemodialysis. One hundred seven patients were randomly assigned to receive intramuscular transplantation of PBMNCs combined with the standard of care (SOC) (cell therapy group; N = 50) or SOC only (SOC group; N = 53). PFS tended to be greater in the cell therapy group compared to the SOC group; however, there was no significant difference (P = 0.07). PFS in Fontaine stage II/III subgroup was significantly better in the cell therapy group than in the control group. The adverse events related to cell therapy were transient and no serious adverse events were observed (Table 1).

Fractionated EPCs (CD34+ Cells)

Phase I/IIa Clinical Studies

Kawamoto et al. conducted a multicenter, single-blinded, dose-escalation phase I/IIa clinical trial of intramuscular transplantation of G-CSF-mobilized CD34+ cells in CLI patients, which started in 2003 in Japan [31]. The study enrolled 17 CLI patients (five with ASO, including one on hemodialysis, and 12 with TAO). The MNCs mobilized by five days of G-CSF treatment were collected by leukapheresis and the CD34+ cells were further isolated using a magnetic-activated cell sorter (CliniMACS®) (Figure 1 and 2). The isolated CD34+ cells, which had a mean purity of 92% and a mean cell viability of 87%, were transplanted to the ischemic lower limbs intramuscularly under lumbar spinal anesthesia (Figure 2).

No death or major amputation of the lower limbs was reported for any patient one year following the treatment. Additionally, all patients maintained independent walking function. The healing of ulcers or necrosis, relief of ischemic pain, and improvement over time with respect to the physiological measures, including TBI and $TcPO_2$ were observed, and 88% of patients were free of CLI one year after the treatment [32]. A long-term follow up over four years following the treatment revealed no deaths in the first two years. Notably, four patients died of cardiac diseases after the first two years; however, a relationship with the cell therapy was ruled out. No major amputation of the lower limbs was reported. The proportion of patients free of CLI remained at over 80% (Figure 3). Significant improvement was noted in TBI at four years and in $TcPO_2$ at three years compared with the pre-treatment data [32].

Ohtake et al. conducted a single-arm, phase II clinical trial of intramuscular transplantation of G-CSF-mobilized CD34+ cells in 6 CLI patients on dialysis [33]. No serious adverse events related to the treatment were reported in the one year following the treatment. The AFS was 100% and 88% of patients were free of CLI one year after the treatment.

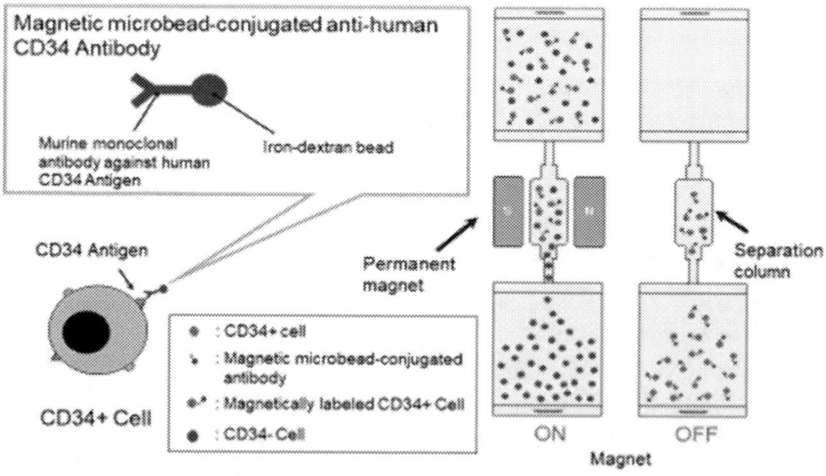

Figure 1. Fundamental principles of the magnetic separation of CD34+ cells.

Table 1. Placebo (or SOC)-controlled, randomized, clinical trials of cell therapy for PAD/CLI

Trial name or author	Phase	Cell type	Route of administration	Disease severity	Cause of PAD	Number of patients	Follow-up duration	Outcomes	
								Primary endpoints	Other endpoints
PROVASA (Walter et al. 2011)	II	Autologous bone marrow mononuclear cells	IA	Rutherford 4-6	ASO TAO	40	3 months	No significant difference in ABI between the cell therapy group and the placebo group.	No significant difference in limb salvage and amputation-free survival rates between the groups. Significant improvement in ulcer area (P = 0.014) and rest pain (P = 0.009) in the cell therapy group compared with the placebo group).
JUVENTUS (Teraa et al. 2015)	II	Autologous bone marrow mononuclear cells	IA	Rutherford 3-6	ASO	160	6 months	No significant difference in the major amputation rate between the cell therapy group and the placebo group.	No significant difference in QOL, rest pain, ABI, and $TcPO_2$ between the groups.
IMPACT (Horie et al. 2018)	III	G-CSF-mobilized autologous peripheral blood mononuclear cells	IM	Fontaine II-IV	ASO TAO	107	1 year	Tendency of improvement in progression-free survival in the cell therapy group compared with the standard of care group (P = 0.07).	In Fontaine II-III, significant improvement in progression-free survival in the cell therapy group compared with the standard of care group. No cell-related safety issues.

Table One. (Continued)

Trial name or author	Phase	Cell type	Route of administration	Disease severity	Cause of PAD	Number of patients	Follow-up duration	Outcomes	
								Primary endpoints	Other endpoints
ACT34-CLI (Losordo et al. 2012)	I/IIa	G-CSF-mobilized autologous peripheral blood CD34+ cells	IM	Rutherford 4-5	ASO TAO	28	1 year	No cell-related safety issues. Reduction of major amputation rate in the cell therapy group compared with the placebo group ($P = 0.125$, at 6 months; $P = 0.058$ at 1 year).	

AFS, amputation-free survival; ASO, arteriosclerosis obliterans; CLI, critical limb ischemia; IA, intra-arterial; IM, intramuscular; PAD, peripheral artery disease; QOL, quality of life; SOC, standard of care: TAO, thromboangiitis obliterans; TBI, toe brachial index.

Tanaka et al. performed a prospective, phase I/IIa clinical trial of G-CSF-mobilized CD34+ cell transplantation for 5 patients with a non-healing diabetic foot [34]. All the enrolled patients were on dialysis. No serious adverse events related to the treatment occurred in one year after the treatment. The wound was completely closed in all the patients at an average of 18 weeks after the treatment.

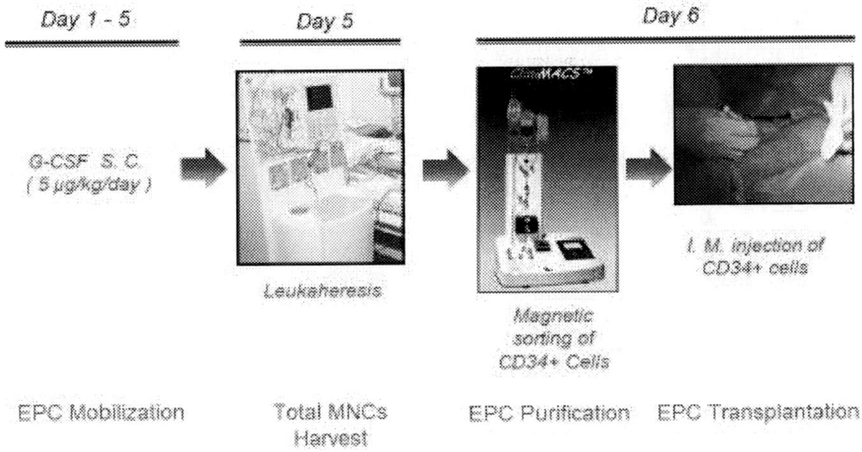

Figure 2. Mobilization, harvesting, isolation, and transplantation of CD34+ cells in CLI patients. EPC, endothelial progenitor cell; G-CSF, granulocyte colony stimulating factor; PBMNC, peripheral blood mononuclear cell.

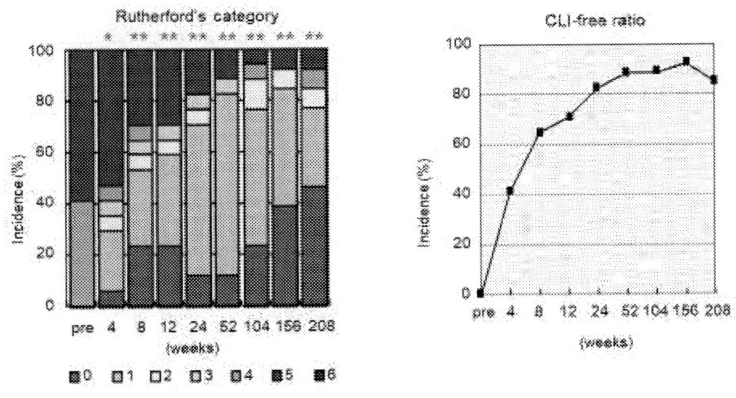

Figure 3. Changes with time in Rutherford's category and the proportion of CLI patients free of CLI within four years after the transplantation of CD34+ cells: results from the Japanese phase I/IIa clinical study.*, $P < 0.05$; **, $P < 0.01$ (compared with pre-transplant); CLI, critical limb ischemia.

In Japan, the G-CSF mobilized CD34+ cell transplantation for CLI patients due to ASO undergoing hemodialysis has been approved as an AMCP-type B since 2017.

In the United States, Losordo et al. initiated a multicenter, randomized, double-blind, placebo-controlled study (ACT34-CLI) in 2007, using the transplantation of G-CSF-mobilized CD34+ cells in 28 patients with CLI caused by ASO [35]. The incidence of minor and major amputations of lower limbs tended to be lower in the CD34+ cell transplantation group than in the placebo group at 6 months (P = 0.125) and 12 months (P = 0.054) after the treatment. No adverse events related to the cell therapy were reported during the one-year follow-up period (Table 1).

In China, Dong et al. compared the therapeutic effect of intramuscular administration of G-CSF-mobilized CD34+ cells with G-CSF-mobilized MNCs in 50 patients with CLI caused by TAO (47 patients) and other angiitis (3 patients) [36]. The CLI patients were randomly assigned (1:1) to receive intramuscular transplantation of G-CSF-mobilized CD34+ cells or G-CSF-mobilized MNCs. The primary efficacy outcomes were major AFS (MAFS) and total AFS (TAFS) rates over 12 months. There were no significant differences in the primary outcome measures of MAFS and TAFS between the CD34+ cell-treated and MNC-treated CLI patients. However, the CD34+ cell-treated patients had a significantly higher probability of rest pain relief than the MNC-treated patients (P = 0.0454).

Investigator-Initiated Study of CD34+ Cell Sorter

Following the early clinical studies described above, an investigator-initiated study in 11 CLI patients (seven with TAO and four with ASO who were not on dialysis) started in 2008 in compliance with good clinical practice for medical devices, aiming a goal of regulatory approval of the CD34+ cell sorter Isolex® [37]. This investigator-initiated study showed favorable safety and efficacy, as had been previously demonstrated in the phase I/IIa study [31, 32] described above. The measures of clinical signs and symptoms, as well as QOL indices, clinical severity, pain at rest, blood flow indices, and walk test results were evaluated frequently. The pain at rest improved soon after the transplantation of CD34+ cells. Physiological improvement was confirmed and improvement in Rutherford's category, the clinical severity index, was demonstrated at approximately 6 months (Figure 4).

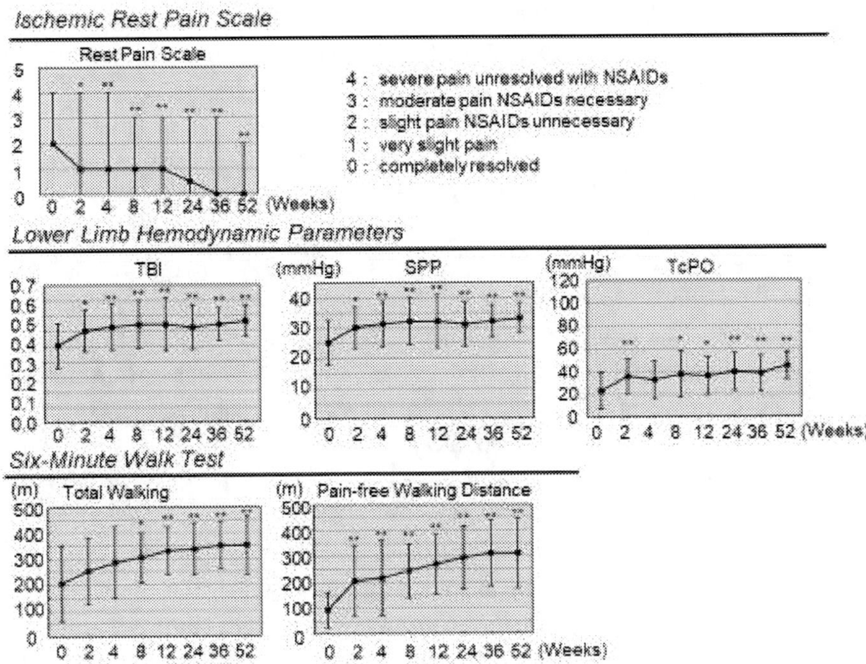

Figure 4. Changes with time with respect to the measures of signs and symptoms up to 52 weeks after the transplantation of CD34+ cells into CLI patients: results from the exploratory investigator-initiated study. SPP, skin perfusion pressure; TBI, toe brachial pressure index; $TcPO_2$, transcutaneous oxygen partial pressure.

Sponsor-Initiated Study Aiming for the Regulatory Approval of CD34+ Cells as a Regenerative-Medicine Product

Furthermore, based on the positive results from the phase I/IIa clinical study [31, 32] and the exploratory investigator-initiated study of the medical device [37], a multicenter, randomized, comparative study in patients with CLI, aiming for regulatory approval of CD34+ cells as a regenerative-medicine product (ClinicalTrials.gov Identifier: NCT02501018) was initiated in December 2017 in Japan, and the first patient was enrolled in the same month. The study is currently ongoing. In March 2018, this regenerative-medicine product was designated by the Ministry of Health, Labor, and Welfare as an appropriate product for the Sakigake Strategy, which consists of the Sakigake Designation System and the Scheme for Rapid Authorization of Unapproved Drugs. This strategy identifies breakthrough medical devices, pharmaceuticals, and regenerative medical products that are designed to treat serious diseases and are likely to be developed first in Japan. Such products are subsequently given priority in consultations and reviews to reduce the review time for approval.

Meta-Analysis of BM-Derived Cell Trials in Patients with CLI

In 2015, Peeters Weem et al. reported a meta-analysis of 10 placebo-controlled, randomized, controlled clinical trials of BM-derived cell therapy in patients with CLI [38]. This meta-analysis studied six clinical trials using BMMNCs, 3 trials using BM-derived mesenchymal stem/stromal cells (MSCs), including Ixmyelocel-T, 1 trial using G-CSF-mobilized CD34+ cells and 1 trial using G-CSF-mobilized CD133+ cells, comparing with placebo-treatment in a total number of 499 patients with CLI (It is notable that one trial was a comparative trial between three groups of BMMNCs, BMMSCs, and placebo). Notably, 80% of the clinical trials analyzed were trials using BMMNCs or BMMSCs. The mean observation period of the trials was 7.5 months, with seven trials reporting 6 months or less of follow up and only three trials with a follow up of 12 months. This meta-analysis demonstrated no significant differences in the primary outcome measures of major amputation rate, survival rate, and AFS between the cell-treated and placebo-treated CLI patients. However, among surrogate outcomes, the wound healing rate in the cell-treated patients tended to be greater (relative risk [RR], 1.40; 95% confidence interval [CI], 0.99–1.97; $P = 0.06$), and ABI ($P < 0.01$), and $TcPO_2$ ($P = 0.01$) and decrease in the rest pain score ($P = 0.03$) in the cell-treated patients were significantly greater compared to the placebo-treated patients.

In 2017, Rigato et al. reported a meta-analysis of 19 randomized, controlled, clinical trials of cell therapy, consisting of 10 placebo-controlled and 9 SOC-controlled trials, and including 837 CLI patients [39]. The cells used for treatment were BMMNCs (9 trials), MSCs (3 trials), Ixmyelocel-T (1 trial), G-CSF-mobilized MNCs (3 trials), G-CSF-mobilized CD34+ cells (1 trial), G-CSF-mobilized CD133+ cells (1 trial), BM concentrate (1 trial), and cultured PB-derived cells (1 trial). One of the 19 trials was a comparative trial between three groups of BMMNCs, BMMSCs, and placebo. Sixty eight percent of the clinical trials analyzed were trials using BMMNCs or BMMSCs. The observation periods of the trials were 22.6 months (1 trial), 12 months (3 trials), and 6 months or less (15 trials). For the primary outcome, cell therapy was associated with a significant 37% reduction in the major amputation rate (RR, 0.63; 95% CI, 0.49–0.82; P = 0.0004), a significant 18% increased probability of AFS (RR, 1.18; 95% CI, 1.04–1.35; P = 0.01) and a significant 59% increased probability of complete wound healing (RR, 1.59; 95% CI, 1.19–2.13; P = 0.002). However, the mortality was not significantly different. Among surrogate outcomes, the cell therapy significantly improved the ABI ($P < .00001$), $TcPO_2$ ($P = .0003$) and reduced the rest pain score ($P = 0.0001$).

The results of these meta-analyses revealed that the effect of cell therapy was controversial with respect to the major amputation rate and AFS, which are common primary outcomes. Additionally, the effect of cell therapy was not shown for survival. On the other hand, the effect of cell therapy was indicated for ABI, $TcPO_2$, and rest pain, which are the surrogate outcomes. However, there are common problems in these meta-analyses. That is, heterogeneity, such as the cell type, route of administration, patient background, severity of limb ischemia, endpoints, and observation period in each clinical trial. In the future, in order to construct stronger evidence for cell therapy, a meta-analysis of the randomized controlled clinical trials that are appropriately designed for specific cell types and administration routes are required.

Conclusion and Future Prospects

Upon summarizing the results of the previous clinical trials in PAD/CLI, EPC therapies may be safe and feasible. Early-phase clinical trials revealed the potential effectiveness of BMMNCs and G-CSF-mobilized PB-MNCs for CLI. However, two randomized, placebo-controlled trials showed no advantage of intraarterial administration of BM-MNCs in CLI patients with ASO with respect to the primary endpoints, ABI and major amputation ratio, respectively (Table 1) [26, 24]. However, BMMNC treatment is expected to be effective for patients with TAO. The results of the clinical trial, which is ongoing as AMCP-type B are awaited. Recently, a culture system to induce EPC-enriched MNCs from unfractionated MNCs has been developed [40]. The development of a cell processing technology may augment the therapeutic potential of MNCs for PAD/CLI. The efficacy and safety of G-CSF-mobilized CD34+ cell therapy has been demonstrated in phase I/II trials. The results of a multicenter, randomized, comparative phase II study in patients with CLI (ClinicalTrials.gov Identifier: NCT02501018), which is ongoing in Japan is expected. Furthermore, the efficacy and safety of CD34+ cell therapy has been demonstrated not only for ischemic diseases such as CLI, refractory angina pectoris [41,42, 43, 44], acute myocardial infarction [45, 46], dilated cardiomyopathy and cerebral infarction [47, 48, 49, 50, 51, 52], but also for nonunion fracture [55] and liver cirrhosis patients [56]. Pharmaceutical approval of CD34+ cells for either of above applications is expected to pave the way for expanding the indication for other diseases.

References

[1] Fowkes F. Gerald R. Rudan Diana, Rudan Igor, Aboyans Victor, Denenberg Julie O. McDermott Mary M. Norman Paul E. Sampson Uchechukwe K. A. Williams Linda J. Mensah George A. and Criqui Michael H. 2013. "Comparison of Global Estimates of Prevalence and Risk Factors for Peripheral Artery Disease in 2000 and 2010: A Systematic Review and Analysis." *Lancet* 382: 1329–40.

[2] Norgren L. Hiatt W. R. Dormandy J. A. Nehler M. R. Harris K. A. Fowkes F. G. and TASC II Working Group. 2007. "Inter-Society Consensus for the Management of Peripheral Arterial Disease (TASC II)." *Journal of Vascular Surgery* 45 Suppl S: S5–67.

[3] Aboyans Victor, Ricco Jean-Baptiste, Bartelink Marie-Louise E. L. Björck Martin, Brodmann Marianne, Cohnert Tina, et. al. 2017. "ESC Guidelines on the Diagnosis and Treatment of Peripheral Arterial Diseases, in Collaboration with the European Society for Vascular Surgery (ESVS)." *European Journal of Vascular and Endovascular Surgery: The Official Journal of the European Society for Vascular Surgery* 55: 305–68.

[4] Fadini Gian Paolo, Agostini Carlo, and Avogaro Angelo. 2010. "Autologous Stem Cell Therapy for Peripheral Arterial Disease Meta-Analysis and Systematic Review of the Literature." *Atherosclerosis* 209: 10–7.

[5] Sprengers R. W. Moll F. L. and Verhaar M. C. 2010. "Stem Cell Therapy in PAD." *European Journal of Vascular and Endovascular Surgery: The Official Journal of the European Society for Vascular Surgery* 39 Suppl 1: S38–43.

[6] Kalka C. Masuda H. Takahashi T. Kalka-Moll W. M. Silver M. Kearney M. Li T. Isner J. M. and Asahara T. 2000. "Transplantation of Ex Vivo Expanded Endothelial Progenitor Cells for Therapeutic Neovascularization." *Proceedings of the National Academy of Sciences of the United States of America* 97: 3422–27.

[7] Murohara T. Ikeda H. Duan J. Shintani S. Sasaki Ki, Eguchi H. Onitsuka I. Matsui K. and Imaizumi T. 2000. "Transplanted Cord Blood-Derived Endothelial Precursor Cells Augment Postnatal Neovascularization." *Journal of Clinical Investigation* 105: 1527–36.

[8] Kawamoto A. Gwon H. C. Iwaguro H. Yamaguchi J. I. Uchida S. Masuda H. Silver M. Ma H. Kearney M. Isner J. M. and Asahara T. 2001. "Therapeutic Potential of Ex Vivo Expanded Endothelial Progenitor Cells for Myocardial Ischemia." *Circulation* 103: 634–37.

[9] Kawamoto Atsuhiko, Iwasaki Hiroto, Kusano Kengo, Murayama Toshinori, Oyamada Akira, Silver Marcy, Hulbert Christine, Gavin Mary, Hanley Allison, Ma Hong, Kearney Marianne, Zak Victor, Asahara Takayuki, and Losordo Douglas W. 2006. "CD34-Positive Cells Exhibit Increased Potency and Safety for Therapeutic Neovascularization after Myocardial Infarction Compared with Total Mononuclear Cells." *Circulation* 114: 2163–9.

[10] Taguchi Akihiko, Soma Toshihiro, Tanaka Hidekazu, Kanda Takayoshi, Nishimura Hiroyuki, Yoshikawa Hiroo, Tsukamoto Yoshitane, Iso Hiroyuki, Fujimori Yoshihiro, Stern David M. Naritomi Hiroaki, and Matsuyama Tomohiro. 2004. "Administration of CD34+ Cells after Stroke Enhances Neurogenesis via Angiogenesis in a Mouse Model." *Journal of Clinical Investigation* 114: 330–8.

[11] Fukui Tomoaki, Mifune Yutaka, Matsumoto Tomoyuki, Shoji Taro, Kawakami Yohei, Kawamoto Atsuhiko, Ii Masaaki, Akimaru Hiroshi, Kuroda Tomoya, Horii Miki, Yokoyama Ayumi, Alev Cantas, Kuroda Ryosuke, Kurosaka Masahiro, and Asahara Takayuki. 2015. "Superior Potential of CD34-Positive Cells Compared to Total Mononuclear Cells for Healing of Nonunion Following Bone Fracture." *Cell Transplantation* 24: 1379–93.

[12] Ii Masaaki, Nishimura Hiromi, Iwakura Atsushi, Wecker Andrea, Eaton Elizabeth, Asahara Takayuki, and Losordo Douglas W. 2005. "Endothelial Progenitor Cells Are Rapidly Recruited to Myocardium and Mediate Protective Effect of Ischemic Preconditioning via 'Imported' Nitric Oxide Synthase Activity." *Circulation* 111: 1114–20.

[13] Jujo Kentaro, Ii Masaaki, and Losordo Douglas W. 2008. "Endothelial Progenitor Cells in Neovascularization of Infarcted Myocardium." *Journal of Molecular and Cellular Cardiology* 45: 530–44.

[14] Miyamoto Yoshiaki, Suyama Takashi, Yashita Tomoko, Akimaru Hiroshi, and Kurata Hirokazu. 2007. "Bone Marrow Subpopulations Contain Distinct Types of Endothelial Progenitor Cells and Angiogenic Cytokine-Producing Cells." *Journal of Molecular and Cellular Cardiology* 43: 627–35.

[15] Sahoo Susmita, Klychko Ekaterina, Thorne Tina, Misener Sol, Schultz Kathryn M. Millay Meredith, Ito Aiko, Liu Ting, Kamide Christine, Agrawal Hemant, Perlman Harris, Qin Gangjian, Kishore Raj, and Losordo Douglas W. 2011. "Exosomes from Human CD34(+) Stem Cells Mediate Their Proangiogenic Paracrine Activity." *Circulation Research* 109: 724–8.

[16] Valadi Hadi, Ekström Karin, Bossios Apostolos, Sjöstrand Margareta, Lee James J. and Lötvall Jan O. 2007. "Exosome-Mediated Transfer of mRNAs and microRNAs is a Novel Mechanism of Genetic Exchange between Cells." *Nature Cell Biology* 9: 654–9.

[17] Yoon Young-Sup, Park Jong-Seon, Tkebuchava Tengiz, Luedeman Corinne, and Losordo Douglas W. 2004. "Unexpected Severe Calcification after Transplantation of Bone Marrow Cells in Acute Myocardial Infarction." *Circulation* 109: 3154–7.

[18] Masuda Haruchika, Alev Cantas, Akimaru Hiroshi, Ito Rie, Shizuno Tomoko, et. al. 2011. "Methodological Development of a Clonogenic Assay to Determine Endothelial Progenitor Cell Potential." *Circulation Research* 109: 20–37.

[19] Tepper Oren M. Galiano Robert D. Capla Jennifer M. Kalka Christoph, Gagne Paul J. Jacobowitz Glen R. Levine Jamie P. and Gurtner Geoffrey C. 2002. "Human Endothelial Progenitor Cells from Type II Diabetics Exhibit Impaired Proliferation, Adhesion, and Incorporation into Vascular Structures." *Circulation* 106: 2781–6.

[20] Vasa M. Fichtlscherer S. Aicher A. Adler K. Urbich C. Martin H. Zeiher A. M. and Dimmeler S. 2001. "Number and Migratory Activity of Circulating Endothelial Progenitor Cells Inversely Correlate with Risk Factors for Coronary Artery Disease." *Circulation Research* 89: E1–7.

[21] Hill Jonathan M. Zalos Gloria, Halcox Julian P. J. Schenke William H. Waclawiw Myron A. Quyyumi Arshed A. and Finkel Toren. 2003. "Circulating Endothelial Progenitor Cells, Vascular Function, and Cardiovascular Risk." *New England Journal of Medicine* 348: 593–600.

[22] Tateishi-Yuyama Eriko, Matsubara Hiroaki, Murohara Toyoaki, Ikeda Uichi, Shintani Satoshi, et. al. 2002. "Therapeutic Angiogenesis for Patients with Limb Ischaemia by Autologous Transplantation of Bone-Marrow Cells: A Pilot Study and a Randomised Controlled Trial." *Lancet* 360: 427–35.

[23] Matoba Satoaki, Tatsumi Tetsuya, Murohara Toyoaki, Imaizumi Tsutomu, Katsuda Yousuke, et. al. 2008. "Long-Term Clinical Outcome after Intramuscular Implantation of Bone Marrow Mononuclear Cells (Therapeutic Angiogenesis by Cell Transplantation [TACT] Trial) in Patients with Chronic Limb Ischemia." *American Heart Journal* 156: 1010–8.

[24] Walter Dirk H. Krankenberg Hans, Balzer J. örn O. Kalka Christoph, Baumgartner Iris, Schlüter Michael, Tonn Torsten, Seeger Florian, Dimmeler Stefanie, Lindhoff-Last Edelgard, Zeiher Andreas M. and PROVASA Investigators. 2011. "Intra-arterial Administration of Bone Marrow Mononuclear Cells in Patients with Critical Limb Ischemia: a Randomized-Start, Placebo-Controlled Pilot Trial (PROVASA)." *Circulation. Cardiovascular Interventions* 4: 26–37.

[25] Powell Richard J. Simons Michael, Mendelsohn Farrel O. Daniel George, Henry Timothy D. Koga Minako, Morishita Ryuichi, and Annex Brian H. 2008. "Results of a Double-Blind, Placebo-Controlled Study to Assess the Safety of Intramuscular Injection of Hepatocyte Growth Factor Plasmid to Improve Limb Perfusion in Patients with Critical Limb Ischemia." *Circulation* 118: 58–65.

[26] Teraa Martin, Sprengers Ralf W., Schutgens Roger E. G., Slaper-Cortenbach Ineke C. M., van der Graaf Yolanda, Algra Ale, van der Tweel Ingeborg, Doevendans Pieter A., Mali Willem P., Th M. Moll Frans L. and Verhaar Marianne C. 2015. "Effect of Repetitive Intra-Arterial Infusion of Bone Marrow Mononuclear Cells in Patients with No-Option Limb Ischemia: The Randomized, Double-Blind, Placebo-Controlled Rejuvenating Endothelial Progenitor Cells via Transcutaneous Intra-Arterial Supplementation (JUVENTAS) Trial." *Circulation* 131: 851–60.

[27] Kondo Kazuhisa, Yanishi Kenji, Hayashida Ryo, Shintani Satoshi, Shibata Rei, Murotani Kenta, Ando Masahiko, Mizuno Masaaki, Fujiwara Tadami, Murohara Toyoaki, Matoba Satoaki, and TACT Follow-up Study Investigators. 2018. "Long-Term Clinical Outcomes Survey of Bone Marrow-Derived Cell Therapy in Critical Limb Ischemia in Japan." *Circulation Journal: Official Journal of the Japanese Circulation Society* 82: 1168–78.

[28] Huang Pingping, Li Shangzhu, Han Mingzhe, Xiao Zhijian, Yang Renchi, and Han Zhong Chao. 2005. "Autologous Transplantation of Granulocyte Colony-Stimulating Factor-Mobilized Peripheral Blood Mononuclear Cells Improves Critical Limb Ischemia in Diabetes." *Diabetes Care* 28: 2155–60.

[29] Ozturk Ahmet, Kucukardali Yasar, Tangi Fatih, Erikci Alev, Uzun Gunalp, Bashekim C. ınar, Sen Huseyin, Terekeci Hakan, Narin Yavuz, Ozyurt Mustafa, Ozkan Sezai, Sayan Ozkan, Rodop Osman, Nalbant Selim, Sıldıroglu Onur, Yalnız Fevzi Firat, Senkal Ibrahim Volkan, Sabuncu Hilmi, and Oktenli Cagatay. 2012. "Therapeutical Potential of Autologous Peripheral Blood Mononuclear Cell Transplantation in Patients with type 2 Diabetic Critical Limb Ischemia." *Journal of Diabetes and its Complications* 26: 29–33.

[30] Horie Takashi, Yamazaki Seiji, Hanada Sayaka, Kobayashi Shuzo, Tsukamoto Tatsuo, et. al. 2018. "Outcome from a Randomized Controlled Clinical Trial-Improvement of Peripheral Arterial Disease by Granulocyte Colony-Stimulating Factor-Mobilized Autologous Peripheral-Blood-Mononuclear Cell Transplantation (IMPACT)." *Circulation Journal: Official Journal of the Japanese Circulation Society* 82: 2165–74.

[31] Kawamoto Atsuhiko, Katayama Minako, Handa Nobuhiro, Kinoshita Makoto, Takano Haruna, et. al. 2009. "Intramuscular Transplanta-tion of G-CSF-Mobilized CD34(+) Cells in Patients with Critical Limb Ischemia: a phase I/IIa, Multicenter, Single-Blinded, Dose-Escalation Clinical Trial." *Stem Cells* 27: 2857–64.

[32] Kinoshita Makoto, Fujita Yasuyuki, Katayama Minako, Baba Rie, Shibakawa Maki, Yoshikawa Kimiko, Katakami Nobuyuki, Furukawa Yutaka, Tsukie Tomio, Nagano Tohru, Kurimoto Yasuo, Yamasaki Kazuo, Handa Nobuhiro, Okada Yukikatsu, Kuronaka Kaori, Nagata Yukiko, Matsubara Yoshihiro, Fukushima Masanori, Asahara Takayuki, and Kawamoto Atsuhiko. 2012. "Long-Term Clinical Outcome after Intramuscular Transplantation of Granulocyte Colony Stimulating Factor-Mobilized CD34 Positive Cells in Patients with Critical Limb Ischemia." *Atherosclerosis* 224: 440–5.

[33] Ohtake Takayasu, Mochida Yasuhiro, Ishioka Kunihiro, Oka Machiko, Maesato Kyoko, Moriya Hidekazu, Hidaka Sumi, Higashide Satoshi, Ioji Tetsuya, Fujita Yasuyuki, Kawamoto Atsuhiko, Fukushima Masanori, and Kobayashi Shuzo. 2018. "Autologous Granulocyte Colony-Stimulating Factor-Mobilized Peripheral Blood CD34 Positive Cell Transplantation for Hemodialysis Patients with Critical Limb Ischemia: a Prospective phase II Clinical Trial." *Stem Cells Translational Medicine* 7: 774–82.

[34] Tanaka Rica, Masuda Haruchika, Kato Shunichi, Imagawa Kotaro, Kanabuchi Kazuo, Nakashioya Chie, Yoshiba Fumiaki, Fukui Tsuyoshi, Ito Rie, Kobori Michiru, Wada Mika, Asahara Takayuki, and Miyasaka Muneo. 2014. "Autologous G-CSF-Mobilized Peripheral Blood CD34+ Cell Therapy for Diabetic Patients with Chronic Nonhealing Ulcer." *Cell Transplantation* 23: 167–79.

[35] Losordo Douglas W. Kibbe Melina R. Mendelsohn Farrell, Marston William, Driver Vickie R. Sharafuddin Melhem, Teodorescu Victoria, Wiechmann Bret N. Thompson Charles, Kraiss Larry, Carman Teresa, Dohad Suhail, Huang Paul, Junge Candice E. Story Kenneth, Weistroffer Tara, Thorne Tina M. Millay Meredith,

Runyon John Paul, Schainfeld Robert, and Autologous CD34+ Cell Therapy for Critical Limb Ischemia Investigators. 2012. "A Randomized, Controlled Pilot Study of Autologous CD34+ Cell Therapy for Critical Limb Ischemia." *Circulation. Cardiovascular Interventions* 5: 821–30.

[36] Dong Zhihui, Pan Tianyue, Fang Yuan, Wei Zheng, Gu Shiyang, Fang Gang, Liu Yifan, Luo Yang, Liu Hao, Zhang Tiejun, Hu Meiyu, Guo Daqiao, Xu Xin, Chen Bin, Jiang Junhao, Yang Jue, Shi Zhenyu, Zhu Ting, Shi Yun, Liu Peng, and Fu Weiguo. 2018. "Purified CD34(+) Cells versus Peripheral Blood Mononuclear Cells in the Treatment of Angiitis-Induced No-Option Critical Limb Ischaemia: 12-Month Results of a Prospective Randomised Single-Blinded Non-Inferiority Trial." *EBiomedicine* 35: 46–57.

[37] Fujita Yasuyuki, Kinoshita Makoto, Furukawa Yutaka, Nagano Tohru, Hashimoto Hisako, Hirami Yasuhiko, Kurimoto Yasuo, Arakawa Kyosuke, Yamazaki Kazuo, Okada Yukikatsu, Katakami Nobuyuki, Uno Emiko, Matsubara Yoshihiro, Fukushima Masanori, Nada Adel, Losordo Douglas W. Asahara Takayuki, Okita Yutaka, and Kawamoto Atsuhiko. 2014. "Phase II Clinical Trial of CD34+ Cell Therapy to Explore Endpoint Selection and Timing in Patients with Critical Limb Ischemia." *Circulation Journal: Official Journal of the Japanese Circulation Society* 78: 490–501.

[38] Peeters Weem S. M. Teraa M. de Borst G. J. Verhaar M. C. and Moll F. L. 2015. "Bone Marrow Derived Cell Therapy in Critical Limb Ischemia: a Meta-Analysis of Randomized Placebo Controlled Trials." *European Journal of Vascular and Endovascular Surgery: the Official Journal of the European Society for Vascular Surgery* 50: 775–83.

[39] Rigato Mauro, Monami Matteo, and Fadini Gian Paolo. 2017. "Autologous Cell Therapy for Peripheral Arterial Disease: Systematic Review and Meta-Analysis of Randomized, Nonrandomized, and Noncontrolled Studies." *Circulation Research* 120: 1326–40.

[40] Masuda Haruchika, Tanaka Rica, Fujimura Satoshi, Ishikawa Masakazu, Akimaru Hiroshi, Shizuno Tomoko, Sato Atsuko, Okada Yoshinori, Iida Yumi, Itoh Jobu, Itoh Yoshiko, Kamiguchi Hiroshi, Kawamoto Atsuhiko, and Asahara Takayuki. 2014. "Vasculogenic Conditioning of Peripheral Blood Mononuclear Cells Promotes Endothelial Progenitor Cell Expansion and Phenotype Transition of Anti-Inflammatory Macrophage and T Lymphocyte to Cells with Regenerative Potential." *Journal of the American Heart Association* 3: e000743.

[41] Henry Timothy D. Losordo Douglas W. Traverse Jay H. Schatz Richard A. Jolicoeur E. Marc, Schaer Gary L. Clare Robert, Chiswell Karen, White Christopher J. Fortuin F. David, Kereiakes Dean J. Zeiher Andreas M. Sherman Warren, Hunt Andrea S. and Povsic Thomas J. 2018. "Autologous CD34+ Cell Therapy Improves Exercise Capacity, Angina Frequency and Reduces Mortality in No-Option Refractory Angina: A Patient-Level Pooled Analysis of Randomized Double-Blinded Trials." *European Heart Journal* 39: 2208–16.

[42] Losordo Douglas W. Henry Timothy D. Davidson Charles, Sup Lee Joon, Costa Marco A. Bass Theodore, Mendelsohn Farrell, Fortuin F. David, Pepine Carl J. Traverse Jay H. Amrani David, Ewenstein Bruce M. Riedel Norbert, Story Kenneth,

Barker Kerry, Povsic Thomas J. Harrington Robert A. Schatz Richard A. and ACT34-CMI Investigators. 2011. "Intramyocardial, Autologous CD34+ Cell Therapy for Refractory Angina." *Circulation Research* 109: 428–36.

[43] Losordo Douglas W., Schatz Richard A., White Christopher J., Udelson James E., Veereshwarayya Vimal, Durgin Michelle, et. al. 2007. "Intramyocardial Transplantation of Autologous CD34+ Stem Cells for Intractable Angina: a phase I/IIa Double-Blind, Randomized Controlled Trial." *Circulation* 115: 3165–72.

[44] Povsic Thomas J., Henry Timothy D., Traverse Jay H. Fortuin F., David, Schaer Gary L., et. al. 2016. "The RENEW Trial: Efficacy and Safety of Intramyocardial Autologous CD34(+) Cell Administration in Patients with Refractory Angina." *JACC. Cardiovascular Interventions* 9: 1576–85.

[45] Quyyumi Arshed A. Vasquez Alejandro, Kereiakes Dean J. Klapholz Marc, Schaer Gary L. Abdel-Latif Ahmed, et. al. 2017. "PreSERVE-AMI: A Randomized, Double-Blind, Placebo-Controlled Clinical Trial of Intracoronary Administration of Autologous CD34+ Cells in Patients with Left Ventricular Dysfunction Post STEMI." *Circulation Research* 120: 324–31.

[46] Quyyumi Arshed A. Waller Edmund K. Murrow Jonathan, Esteves Fabio, Galt James, Oshinski John, Lerakis Stamatios, Sher Salman, Vaughan Douglas, Perin Emerson, Willerson James, Kereiakes Dean, Gersh Bernard J. Gregory Douglas, Werner Astrid, Moss Thomas, Chan Wai Shun, Preti Robert, and Pecora Andrew L. 2011. "CD34(+) Cell Infusion after ST Elevation Myocardial Infarction is Associated with Improved Perfusion and is Dose Dependent." *American Heart Journal* 161: 98–105.

[47] Bervar Mojca, Kozelj Mirta, Poglajen Gregor, Sever Matjaz, Zemljic Gregor, Frljak Sabina, Cukjati Marko, Cernelc Peter, Haddad François, and Vrtovec Bojan. 2017. "Effects of Transendocardial CD34(+) Cell Transplantation on Diastolic Parameters in Patients with Nonischemic Dilated Cardiomyopathy." *Stem Cells Translational Medicine* 6: 1515–21.

[48] Frljak Sabina, Jaklic Martina, Zemljic Gregor, Cerar Andraz, Poglajen Gregor, and Vrtovec Bojan. 2018. "CD34(+) Cell Transplantation Improves Right Ventricular Function in Patients with Nonischemic Dilated Cardiomyopathy." *Stem Cells Translational Medicine* 7: 168–72.

[49] Lezaic Luka, Socan Aljaz, Poglajen Gregor, Peitl Petra Kolenc, Sever Matjaz, Cukjati Marko, Cernelc Peter, Wu Joseph C. Haddad François, and Vrtovec Bojan. 2015. "Intracoronary Transplantation of CD34+ Cells Is Associated with Improved Myocardial Perfusion in Patients with Nonischemic Dilated Cardiomyopathy." *Journal of Cardiac Failure* 21: 145–52.

[50] Vrtovec Bojan, Poglajen Gregor, Lezaic Luka, Sever Matjaz, Domanovic Dragoslav, Cernelc Peter, Socan Aljaz, Schrepfer Sonja, Torre-Amione Guillermo, Haddad François, and Wu Joseph C. 2013. "Effects of Intracoronary CD34+ Stem Cell Transplantation in Nonischemic Dilated Cardiomyopathy Patients: 5-Year Follow-Up." *Circulation Research* 112: 165–73.

[51] Vrtovec Bojan, Poglajen Gregor, Lezaic Luka, Sever Matjaz, Socan Aljaz, Domanovic Dragoslav, Cernelc Peter, Torre-Amione Guillermo, Haddad François, and Wu Joseph C. 2013. "Comparison of Transendocardial and Intracoronary

CD34+ Cell Transplantation in Patients with Nonischemic Dilated Cardiomyopathy." *Circulation* 128 Suppl 1: S42–9.

[52] Vrtovec Bojan, Poglajen Gregor, Sever Matjaz, Lezaic Luka, Domanovic Dragoslav, Cernelc Peter, Haddad François, and Torre-Amione Guillermo. 2011. "Effects of Intracoronary Stem Cell Transplantation in Patients with Dilated Cardiomyopathy." *Journal of Cardiac Failure* 17: 272–81.

[53] Banerjee Soma, Bentley Paul, Hamady Mohammad, Marley Stephen, Davis John, Shlebak Abdul, Nicholls Joanna, Williamson Deborah A. Jensen Steen L. Gordon Myrtle, Habib Nagy, and Chataway Jeremy. 2014. "Intra-Arterial Immunoselected CD34+ Stem Cells for Acute Ischemic Stroke." *Stem Cells Translational Medicine* 3: 1322–30.

[54] Chen Der-Cherng, Lin Shinn-Zong, Fan Jia-Rong, Lin Chen-Huan, Lee Wei, Lin Chao-Chun, Liu Yi-Jui, Tsai Chon-Haw, Chen Jui-Cheng, Cho Der-Yan, Lee Chau-Chin, and Shyu Woei-Cherng. 2014. "Intracerebral Implantation of Autologous Peripheral Blood Stem Cells in Stroke Patients: A Randomized phase II Study." *Cell Transplantation* 23: 1599–612.

[55] Kuroda Ryosuke, Matsumoto Tomoyuki, Niikura Takahiro, Kawakami Yohei, Fukui Tomoaki, Lee Sang Yang, Mifune Yutaka, Kawamata Shin, Fukushima Masanori, Asahara Takayuki, Kawamoto Atsuhiko, and Kurosaka Masahiro. 2014. "Local Transplantation of Granulocyte Colony Stimulating Factor-Mobilized CD34+ Cells for Patients with Femoral and Tibial Nonunion: Pilot Clinical Trial." *Stem Cells Translational Medicine* 3: 128–34.

[56] Nakamura Toru, Torimura Takuji, Iwamoto Hideki, Kurogi Jyunichi, Inoue Hiroto, Hori Yukie, Sumie Shuji, Fukushima Nobuyoshi, Sakata Masahiro, Koga Hironori, Abe Mitsuhiko, Ikezono Y. Hashimoto Osamu, Ueno Takato, Oho Kazuhiko, Okamura Takashi, Okuda Seiya, Kawamoto Atsuhiko, Ii Masaaki, Asahara Takayuki, and Sata Michio. 2014. "CD34(+) Cell Therapy Is Safe and Effective in Slowing the Decline of Hepatic Reserve Function in Patients with Decompensated Liver Cirrhosis." *Journal of Gastroenterology and Hepatology* 29: 1830–8.

Chapter 7

EPC in Kidney Disease

Takayasu Ohtake[1,2,3,*],
and Shuzo Kobayashi[2,3], MD, PhD
[1]Regenerative Medicine, Center for Cell Therapy and Regenerative Medicine,
Shonan Kamakura General Hospital, Kamakura, Japan
[2]Shonan Research Institute of Innovative Medicine,
Shonan Kamakura General Hospital, Kamakura, Japan
[3]Kidney and Transplant Center,
Shonan Kamakura General Hospital, Kamakura, Japan

Abstract

Acute and chronic kidney injury is a major and spreading public health problem in the world, not only because of its high prevalence and ultimate progression to end-stage renal failure (ESRD), but because of the high morbidity and mortality associated with cardiovascular diseases. Despite the recent progression of treatment strategies, including an effective pharmacological approach, there has been no established treatment to sufficiently retard or improve the progressive deterioration of kidney dysfunction.

Preclinical studies and recent clinical trials have demonstrated evidence of the efficacy of stem/progenitor cell-based therapy for several disease conditions, which are refractory to present treatment strategies. Recently, regenerative medicine has been extensively investigated and has emerged as a state-of-the-art medicine. Among the cells used for cell therapy, endothelial progenitor cells (EPCs), derived from hematopoietic stem cells (HSCs) in the bone marrow, has a variety of beneficial actions as a tool for regenerative therapy.

---

* Corresponding Author's Email: ohtake@shonankamakura.or.jp.

In: Endothelial Progenitor Cells in Health and Disease
Editors: Amankeldi A. Salybekov, Shuzo Kobayashi and Takayuki Asahara
ISBN: 978-1-68507-794-5

Recent advances elucidated that microcirculatory impairment in the kidney due to acute or chronic ischemia/hypoxia is one of the major causes of kidney dysfunction, leading to permanent damages to the glomerulus, tubulus, and interstitium, both in acute and chronic kidney disease. The integrity of microcirculation, especially integrity in glomerular and peritubular capillary endothelial cells, is shown to be the most important target for regenerative therapy in kidney disease. The suppression of inflammation and interstitial fibrosis are also important targets for the repair of renal tissue. In this setting, it seems reasonable to apply EPCs, with its strong angiogenic and anti-inflammatory actions, for kidney disease.

Keywords: acute kidney injury, chronic kidney disease, CD34, endothelial, progenitor cell, angiogenesis

Introduction

Because of the high prevalence and strong impact on mortality, both acute kidney injury (AKI) and chronic kidney disease (CKD) are regarded as one of the major devastating diseases in humans. In AKI, there has still been no established treatment to effectively improve acute renal dysfunction. In CKD, although several treatments including blood pressure control, diet control, renin-angiotensin-aldosterone system (RAAS) blockade, and metabolic control are provided, these treatments have still not yet achieved sufficient results to inhibit or retard the progression of CKD. Therefore, several patients with kidney disease ultimately progress to end-stage renal failure (ESRD).

The kidney has a very complex and delicate structure composed of several components including the glomerulus, tubulus, interstitium, and vasculature. The kidney parenchyma is composed of the cortex and medulla; additionally, the medulla is separated into the outer and inner medulla with different roles and functions. The glomerulus is composed of glomerular epithelial cells (podocytes), endothelial cells, and mesangial cells, and the tubulus is composed of proximal tubulus, ascending and descending limb, Henle-loop, distal tubulus, and collecting ducts. Post-glomerular peritubular capillaries (PTCs) surround these tubules in a complex manner to deliver oxygen and nutrients to these cells. The interstitium supports these complex structures. Therefore, the established renal structural damages, such as glomerulo-sclerosis and/or interstitial fibrosis have been previously believed not to regress or restore. However, in the recent decades, we came to understand a fact that renal structural damages could be restored. In animal models of kidney disease, the angiotensin receptor blockade caused remodeling of glomerular sclerosis in aging rats [1, 2]; additionally, aldosterone inhibition regressed existing glomeruloscerosis in 5/6 nephrectomized rats [3]. Notable direct evidence for the regeneration of renal injury in human was first reported by Fiorreto et al. in 1998 [4]. They found that the changes of diabetic nephropathy were reversed after pancreatic transplantation in type 1 diabetic patients, although 10 years after transplantation were necessary. Mesangial matrix expansion was significantly decreased at 10 years after transplantation (normalization of glucose metabolism) compared with that of the baseline and 5 years after transplantation.

We also confirmed the regenerative potential of the damaged structures in the kidney. Angiotensin type 1 receptor blocker (ARB) monotherapy showed pathological regression in patients with mesangial proliferative glomerulonephritis [5]. A repeated renal biopsy was performed after a mean of 28.1 months, and the mesangial matrix expansion and interstitial fibrosis rates were significantly reduced compared with those at baseline. Therefore, damaged structures in the human kidney could be restored even though a long time might be necessary.

Tissue repair depends on the balance between the severity of damage and the regenerative potential. Organ damage also depends on the time course of injury, i.e. acute or chronic injury. If the damage is weak enough for restoration, the damage could be restored. However, acute severe damage and/or chronic continuous damage, which exceeds the regenerative capacity, would lead to permanent unrepairable organ damages. For support and promotion of the regenerative process, cell-based therapy has emerged and now has been applied in several diseases. Somatic stem cells, including $CD34^+$ endothelial progenitor cells (EPCs) or mesenchymal stem cells (MSCs), have mainly been used as the sources of regenerative therapy in kidney disease. In this chapter, we review the pathophysiology of kidney disease, implication of EPC in kidney disease, and the efficacy of $CD34^+$ EPCs in preclinical animal studies and clinical trials for AKI and CKD in human kidney disease.

Pathophysiology of Kidney Disease

CKD is a progressive disease leading to ESRD with increasing incidence and mortality [6]. Renal parenchymal diseases are broadly divided into glomerular disease, vascular disease, and tubulointerstitial disease. Injuries in the glomerulus, vessels, and tubulointerstitium mutually influence and form a vicious cycle to worsen the kidney function. Regardless of the initial causes, a continuous decrease of the glomerular filtration rate (GFR) leads several CKD patients to ESRD. In this situation, tubular atrophy and interstitial fibrosis rather than the injury in the glomerulus correlated with renal function [7]; additionally, tubulointerstitial damage is an important final common pathway leading to ESRD [8, 9].

Microvasculature loss and tissue hypoxia are characteristic features in progressive kidney disease [10] and forms a close association with interstitial fibrosis [11, 12]. Hypoxic stimuli to tubular epithelial cells increase the synthesis of the extracellular matrix and type 1 collagen and decreases the collagenase activity and turnover of renal fibroblasts [12]. Furthermore, hypoxia induces interstitial fibrosis via accelerated fibrogenesis by interstitial fibroblasts [12]. Hypoxia is also a potent stimulus for the recruitment of inflammatory cells, such as macrophages and T lymphocytes, which produce profibrotic cytokines, such as TGF-β1. The post-glomerular capillary flow is essential for the delivery of oxygen and nutrients to the tubulointerstitium [10, 13]. The obsolescence of the glomerular capillary leads to a decreased blood supply of downstream PTC, leading to tubular and interstitial hypoxia. However, it is shown that tubulointerstitial injury occurs prior to a development of glomerulosclerosis through a decrease in the postglomerular capillary blood flow [14]. Fibrosis increases the diffusion distance between the functional vessels and nephrons, exacerbating the hypoxia. Interstitial fibrosis also increases the PTC pressure, thus leading to reduced PTC flow and exaggerates the tubular epithelial hypoxia. PTC loss, reduced postglomerular capillary flow, is shown in progressive kidney disease, and a reduced blood supply plays an essential and pivotal role as an etiology of interstitial fibrosis [13].

Although up to 25% of blood volume ejected from the heart entry to the kidney, blood distribution in the kidney is not homogeneous. Blood supply is much more in the cortex than in the medullary region to secure sufficient blood volume for glomerular filtration and for the workload of the reabsorption of solutes. The average partial oxygen pressure in the renal cortex is 30 ~ 50 mmHg, and 10 mmHg (normally as low as 4 ~ 5 mmHg) in the medulla [15]. Especially, the outer medulla forms a countercurrent system, and oxygen escape from the artery to the vein (arterial to venous diffusional oxygen shunt) occurs [16, 17]. Furthermore, the oxygen demand is very high in the S3 segment of proximal tubules and thick ascending limb (TAL) in the outer stripe of the outer medulla (OSOM) due to workload of active sodium transport (increased Na^+/K^+-ATPase activity). An increase in the workload due to sodium transport induces cell hypertrophy with an upregulation of insulin-like growth factor and insulin-like growth factor binding proteins, suggesting that an increased oxygen demand in the tubular epithelial cells plays an important role for renal injury [18]. Therefore, the influence of ischemia (hypoxia) first occurs in the outer medulla. A prolonged reduction of medullary blood flow has been reported in the ischemia/reperfusion AKI model [19]. The medullary blood flow was still reduced 1 ~ 2 hours after reperfusion, when the cortex blood flow recovered normally [20-22]. These ischemic damages induced capillary endothelial injury, leading to peritubular capillary rarefaction, further damaging tubular and interstitial cells. The continuous or prolonged reduction of blood supply in the outer medulla both in acute and chronic kidney injury exaggerates the damage of tubular epithelial cells, especially S3 segment proximal tubular epithelial cells in the outer medulla. Incomplete or failed recovery from AKI leads to long-term functional deficits (AKI to CKD transition) [23]. De-differentiated tubular epithelial cells during regeneration after IRI exhibit persistent, unregulated, and increasing profibrotic signaling. Paracrine products from these tubular epithelial cells damage normal interaction between the PTC endothelium and fibroblasts adjacent to PTC, leading to myofibroblast transformation, proliferation, and fibrosis as well as capillary disintegration and rarefaction. A part of the proximal tubular epithelial cells, that dedifferentiate during regeneration after IRI, fail to re-differentiate and regain the normal tubular structure during recovery. Tubulointerstitial damage was shown to emerge as late as several months after ischemia/reperfusion AKI [24]. Acute ischemic renal injury results in permanent damage to PTC and influences the long-term function.

Renal erythropoietin-producing cells (REPs) produce erythropoietin (EPO), red blood cell producing hormone, according to hypoxic stimuli and/or anemia [25]. The hematopoietic function of REPs is thought to be mediated by the O_2-sensing mechanism of these cells. The origin of REPs is renal fibroblasts, which are located in the peritubular interstitial space around PTC [26-29]. Under hypoxic stimuli, REPs transdifferentiate into myofibroblast and predominantly contribute to fibrosis along with attenuated erythropoietin production [30]. The finding by Norman et al. [12] that interstitial fibroblasts accelerate the fibrotic process in response to hypoxia was confirmed by more precise evaluations of the fibroblast-to-myofibroblast trans-differentiation in hypoxic circumstances [30].

Angiotensin II is an important substance, which regulates the blood pressure and sodium reabsorption. Angiotensin II promotes vascular endothelial cell dysfunction, smooth muscle cell proliferation, and inflammation via the production of reactive oxygen species (ROS) from vascular smooth muscle cells [31], leading to the progression of atherosclerosis and chronic kidney dysfunction. Angiotensin II also regulates the renal medullary blood flow via the production of nitric oxide and ROS. Additionally, angiotensin II is known to induce tubulointerstitial injury with phenotypic changes [32]. Kobayashi et al. provided evidence stating that ARB improved tubulointerstitial injury in animal models of kidney disease by the inhibition of phenotypic changes in tubulointerstitial cells [33, 34]. Tubulointerstitial cells acquired new smooth muscle cell and fibroblastic characteristics associated with the neo-expression of cytoplasmic cytoskeletal proteins (α smooth muscle actin and vimentin) in 5/6 nephrectomy rats and 2-kidney, 1-clip Goldblatt hypertensive rats. The ARB significantly improved tubulointerstitial injury associated with the improvement of myofibroblastic phenotypic changes [33, 34]. Thus, angiotensin II is an important mediator for the progression of tubulointerstitial injury.

Vascular endothelial growth factor (VEGF) is a major proangiogenic cytokine released from ischemic tissue in response to hypoxic stimuli. VEGF is a proliferative-, survival-, and trophic-factor of the vascular endothelial cells [35]. VEGF increases the endothelial nitric oxide synthase (eNOS) activity via VEGFR2. VEGF is constitutively expressed in the normal kidney. Additionally, its expression is primarily localized to the glomerular podocyte, and to tubular cells, especially in the outer medulla and medullary rays [36]. A decreased expression of VEGF closely correlates with PTC loss and tubulointerstitial inflammation [37]. Hypoxia induces the inflammatory cell infiltration [38]. The cytokines released from infiltrated macrophages, including interleukin (IL) -1β, tumor necrosis factor (TNF) -α, and IL-6, in turn, inhibited VEGF mRNA and protein expression in medullary TAL. Externally administered VEGF improved the renal function and capillary loss in Thy1.1 glomerulonephritis and 5/6 nephrectomy model [39, 40]. Glomerular capillary repair was induced by VEGF administration. Progressive renal disease was associated with loss of the glomerular and peritubular capillary microvasculature, and this has been associated with defective capillary repair due in part to an imbalance in the renal expression of angiogenic VEGF and antiangiogenic thrombospondin-1 [10]. As shown in Table 1, a variety of angiogenic and antiangiogenic factors are known to influence the endothelial cell integrity. The pathophysiology for progressive renal disease is summarized in Figure 1.

Table 1. Endogenous factors that modulate endothelial cell integrity

Proangiogenic factors	Antiangiogenic factors
Vascular endothelial growth factor (VEGF)	Thrombospondin-1
Basic fibroblast growth factor (bFGF)	Angiostatin
Hepatocyte growth factor (HGF)	Endostatin
Prostaglandin E2 (PGE2)	
Angiopoietin	

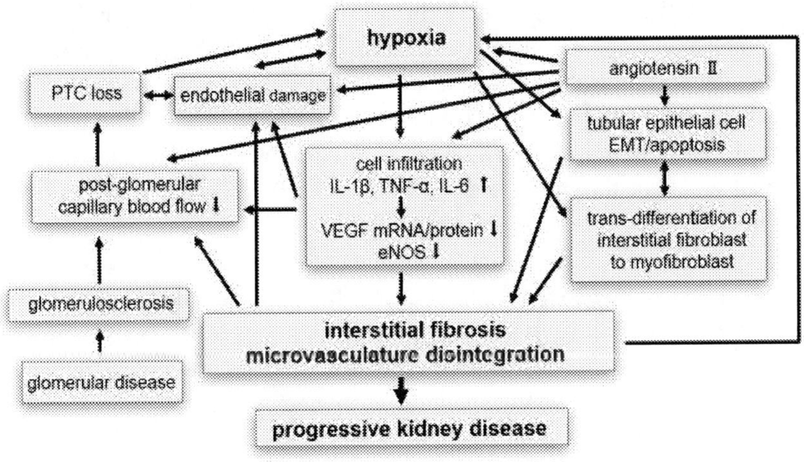

Figure 1. Pathophysiology of progressive kidney disease. Hypoxia and subsequent interstitial fibrosis (caused by inflammatory cell infiltration, tubular epithelial cell apoptosis/EMT, interstitial fibroblast transdifferentiation to myofibroblast) induce PTC rarefaction and destruction of microvascular integrity, leading to progressive kidney disease. Abbreviations: EMT = epithelial-mesenchymal transition; EPO = erythropoietin; PTC = peritubular capillary; IL = interleukin; TNF= tumor necrosis factor; VEGF= vascular endothelial growth factor.

EPC in Kidney Disease

EPC Count and Function in Kidney Disease

CKD patients are at a great risk of cardiovascular events and mortality, and the risk increases with the progression of kidney disease [41]. CKD accelerates atherosclerosis, which promotes ischemic heart disease, heart failure, cerebrovascular disease, and peripheral artery disease [42-46]. The most important characteristics of atherosclerosis in CKD patients are accelerated endothelial dysfunction [47, 48] and vascular calcification [49, 50], both of which concomitantly leads to so-called "vascular failure" [51, 52]. The vascular endothelial cells have several important biological actions on vascular homeostasis, including angiogenesis, hemodynamics, immunological reaction, vasomotor tone control, membrane permeability, and anti-thrombosis. The dysfunction of vascular endothelial cells leads to the failure of these important regulating mechanisms. Vascular endothelial cell dysfunction is an initial step of atherosclerosis and is found even in the early stage of CKD [53]. In case of endothelial dysfunction, EPC functions as an endogenous agent for repairing the vascular endothelium, contributing to angiogenesis, and retards the progression of atherosclerosis.

EPCs exist in the bone marrow, and the number of circulating EPCs in peripheral blood is very low (0.01% of mononuclear cells). Normally, the number of EPCs in the peripheral blood is 5 ~ 40 cells/mm^3 [54]. However, the number of EPCs in the peripheral blood is significantly decreased in patients with CKD [47, 55-62]. The number of circulating EPCs is clinically very important because they might represent the potential of endothelial repair and angiogenic function. Indeed, low circulating CD34$^+$ cells count was significantly correlated with poor prognoses in hemodialysis patients. Low circulating EPCs count was associated with poor cardiovascular event-free survival and all-cause survival [63].

The decrease of CD34+ EPCs was shown even in the early stage of CKD, and more prominent along with the progression of CKD stage [56]. A strong inverse association between the number of circulating EPCs and glomerular filtration ratio (GFR) was reported [57], and the most prominent decrease in circulating CD34+ EPCs was shown in dialysis patients [47, 55-63]. CD34+/CD133+ EPCs showed significant inverse correlation with the serum levels of uremic toxin, indole-3-acetic acid, and uremia-associated parameter β 2 microglobulin [47].

CKD not only influences the number of circulating EPCs, but also strongly affects its angiogenic and proliferating function [55, 56, 62]. The serum of uremic patients inhibited the differentiation, migration, and outgrowth of EPCs [55, 56]. The culture of EPCs with urea accelerated the synthesis of reactive oxygen species (ROS), subsequently reducing the EPC colony-forming unit and inhibited the differentiation to CD31$^+$ and VEGFR2$^+$ cells [62].

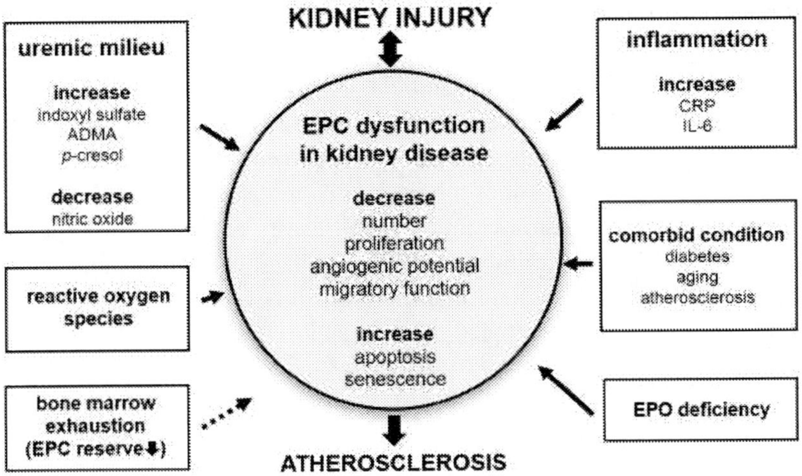

Figure 2. Causative factors for EPC dysfunction in kidney disease. Several factors simultaneously contribute to EPC dysfunction in patients with kidney disease. Abbreviations: ADMA = asymmetric dimethylarginine; CRP = C-reactive protein; IL = interleukin; EPO = erythropoietin.

The decrease of circulating EPCs count might be derived from a variety of causative factors including the reduction of EPCs reserve in the bone marrow, mobilization defect from bone marrow, survival shortening, and reduced proliferating potential. "Bone marrow exhaustion," a severe reduction of the stem/progenitor cell reserve in the bone marrow, might be also associated in patients with ESRD, as is reported in patients with critical limb threatening ischemia (CLTI) [64]. Erythropoietin (EPO) deficiency in CKD also mediates the number and function of EPCs [65, 66]. EPO deficiency was correlated with the decrease in the circulating EPCs number; additionally, the administration of erythropoiesis-stimulating agents (ESA) increased the number and cell activity (increased cell proliferation) of EPCs. *eNOS* is essential for the mobilization of EPCs [67]. However, the plasma levels of endogenous *eNOS* inhibitor, asymmetric dimethylarginine, is elevated in CKD patients [68]. Microinflammation (elevation of C-reactive protein, interleukin-6, etc.) induced under uremic milieu is also associated with EPC dysfunction. Inflammation induces EPC senescence and apoptosis [69-72]. The plasma levels of indoxyl sulfate (IS), one of the major uremic toxins, which accumulates in the blood in cases of kidney dysfunction, was inversely correlated with the number of circulating EPCs [73]. IS is a protein-bound uremic toxin, and therefore not cleared by dialysis. IS levels are known to be a strong predictor of mortality and cardiovascular events in CKD patients [74]. The IS levels also closely correlate with the microcirculatory impairment in CKD patients [75]. IS lowering treatment by AST-120, an oral charcoal adsorbent of IS precursor indole in the gastrointestinal tract, significantly improved the microcirculatory impairment represented as skin perfusion pressure (SPP) [75]. In the hindlimb ischemia model in subtotal nephrectomized mice, AST-120 administration significantly reversed the impaired neovascularization in the hindlimb via EPCs mobilization and vascular repair [76]. The causative factors, which influence on the number and function of circulating EPCs in patients with CKD are shown in Figure 2.

Response of EPC to Kidney Injury

The renal microvasculature plays a pivotal role in the maintenance of the normal renal function. Additionally, the integrity of the vascular endothelium is very important to maintain the function of the microvasculature. In cases of endothelial injury, EPCs contribute to microvascular repair. Hohenstein et al. investigated the response of EPCs in selective unilateral endothelial injury of the mouse kidney [77]. Selective endothelial injury in the kidney induced a marked stimulation of EPCs, and various angiogenic factors orchestrate the microvascular repair. A rise in the EPCs in the peripheral blood was detected as early as 3 hours after disease induction and persisted for 3 days. The surge in EPCs was restricted in the injured kidney, and contralateral kidney showed no increase in EPCs, indicating specific homing factors in injured tissue. Along with EPCs mobilization, a large variety of chemokines and angiogenic factors were involved in the response to endothelial injury. The angiogenic factors started to increase as early as 30 min after disease induction. The first and most significant increase occurred in MMP-9 levels, followed by the subsequent increase in IL-6, TNF-α, IL-10, granulocyte colony-stimulating factor (G-CSF), and granulocyte macrophage colony-stimulating factor (GM-CSF). These angiogenic factors are released upon endothelial injury, and potentially contribute to inflammatory response or the early induction of protective and/or repair mechanisms.

EPC Therapy for Kidney Disease

Basic Research

Despite the elucidation of major factors involved in AKI and CKD, and development of better treatments, the number of individuals with ESRD is steadily increasing. Preclinical studies have suggested the beneficial effects of cell-based therapy in AKI and CKD, although this has not yet been fully translated to the clinical setting. Here, we present the findings of preclinical studies using EPCs or EPC products (EVs) on animal models of AKI and CKD, and proposed mechanisms for their efficacy.

AKI

Unilateral or bilateral ischemia/reperfusion injury (IRI) in the mouse or rat is frequently used for AKI induction (Table 2). One important issue in the repair dynamics of damaged organs is whether acute ischemia induces the mobilization of EPCs from the bone marrow and aids in homing them to the injured tissue. Patschan et al. have clearly elucidated this issue. The acute ischemic signal in the kidney promptly stimulated the mobilization and homing of EPCs [78]. Increased numbers of EPCs were first shown in the spleen at 3 and 6 hours after IRI; additionally, splenectomy before IRI induced the surge of circulating EPCs. During the 7 days after IRI, EPCs were accumulated and were localized mainly in the medullo-papillary region in the kidney.

Table 2. Efficacy of EPCs or EPC product (EVs) on AKI in animal models

Author And Year	Animal	Model	Cell Type	Efficacy
Patchan D (2006)	Mouse	IRI	Mouse EPC	Yes
Dekel B (2006)	Mouse	IRI	Human EPC	Yes
Li B (2010)	Mouse	IRI	Human PBEPC	Yes
Cantaluppi V (2012)	Rat	IRI	Human PBEPC-EV	Yes
Li L (2012)	Mouse	IRI	Mouse PBEPC	Yes
Burger D (2015)	Mouse	IRI	Human UCBEPC/Evs	Yes
Ohtake T (2018)	Mouse	IRI	Human Qqc-PBMNC	Yes

As for the efficacy of human EPCs, EPCs derived from peripheral blood (PB) and/or umbilical cord blood (UCB) significantly inhibited the progression of AKI [79-84]. These studies excellently indicated the efficacy of human EPCs on AKI induced by IRI. Histological findings, including acute tubular necrosis, inflammatory cell infiltration, necrosis and/or apoptosis of tubular epithelial cells were significantly improved by the administration of EPCs. However, almost all studies administered cells at the induction or shortly after the induction of IRI, focusing on the primary prevention of AKI [79, 81-83]. However, in consideration of clinical AKI, a lot of patients have pre-established severe AKI before treatment. Therefore, the evaluation of the efficacy of cell-based therapy in preestablished AKI is important in preclinical studies. Li et al. and we found and reported the efficacy of human EPC-enriched cell fraction on preestablished severe AKI, respectively [80, 84]. Li et al. and the present authors administered cells at 24 hours after IRI induction, at which time severe AKI has already been established. Li et al. used mobilized human PBEPCs, and we used human PB-derived cultured mononuclear cells (PBMNCs). The PBMNCs were obtained from healthy volunteers, and preincubated in a vasculogenic conditioning medium (quality and quantity control culture: QQc-culture) for 7 days before the administration. QQc-culture is an established and excellent method to enhance the number and proliferating potential of $CD34^+$ EPCs [85]. Notably, QQc-culture not only significantly increased the number of $CD34^+$ EPCs, but also dramatically changed the proportion of macrophages (inflammatory M1 and reparative M2). One week's culture of PBMNCs remarkably increased the $CD206^+$ M2 macrophages along with the decrease in M1 macrophages, leading to a significantly decreased M1/M2 ratio. Thus, the component of QQc-cultured PBMNCs was enriched in proangiogenic $CD34^+$ EPCs and anti-inflammatory M2 macrophages. The transplantation of these cells significantly improved the renal function and renal histological injuries 48 hours after cell administration [84]. Although engraftment of human cells in the intracapillary lumen or interstitial space just around PTCs was rather rare compared to the accumulation in the lung or spleen, the improvement of AKI was accompanied by better preservation of PTCs, thus suggesting the important role of integrity of PTC network and protective effect of EPCs on vascular endothelial cells (Figure 3).

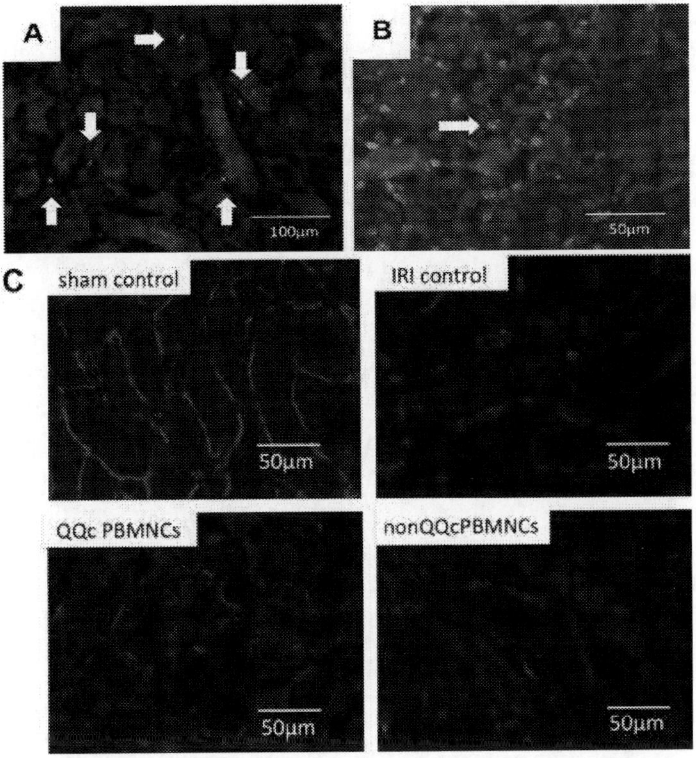

Figure 3. Homing of transplanted human cells and improvement of PTC rarefaction in IRI. (A) Cell tracker-labeled green-colored human QQc-cultured PBMNCs are seen in the space between tubules (arrow) 24 hours after cell transplantation. (B) Cell tracker-labeled green-colored human QQc-cultured PBMNCs cells were located in the inner space of PTCs adjacent to the capillary wall (arrow). (C) CD31 immunofluorescent staining of kidney sections of sham control, IRI control, QQc PBMNCs, and non-QQc PBMNCs at 48 hours after IRI induction (24 hours after cell transplantation). EPC-enriched QQc-cultured PBMNCs significantly improved PTC loss compared with IRI control. Non-QQc cultured PBMNCs did not improve PTC loss. *Abbreviations: QQc = quality and quantity control; PBMNC = peripheral blood mononuclear cells; PTC = peritubular capillary; IRI = ischemia/reperfusion injury; EPC = endothelial progenitor cell.*

CKD

Anti-Thy1.1 glomerulonephritis, 5/6 nephrectomy, renal artery stenosis, and db/db genetic type 2 diabetic nephropathy were used as the CKD models for the evaluation of efficacy of cell therapy (Table 3) [86-94]. Anti-Thy1.1

glomerulonephritis is an established model of mesangial and glomerular endothelial cell injury. By administering a complement-fixing antibody to Thy1 antigen present on the mesangial cell membrane, acute mesangial cell loss and matrix dissolution, ballooning of glomerular capillaries, subsequent formation of microaneurysm and loss of endothelial cells could be induced [95]. Using this model, Rookmaaker et al. provided an important finding stating that the repair of glomerular injury involves BM-derived cells [96]. Allogeneic rat BM cells transplanted to rats with anti-Thy1.1 glomerulonephritis significantly engrafted into the injured glomerulus and repaired glomerular injuries by transdifferentiating to the mesangial and endothelial cells. BM-derived cells participated in the glomerular endothelial and mesangial cell turnover and contributed to microvascular repair. Subsequently, Uchimura et al. provided exogenously administered rat culture-modified BM cells, cultured in the medium promoting EPCs growth, significantly improved glomerular injury, macrophage infiltration, and decrease in the glomerular endothelial cells in anti-Thy1.1 glomerulonephritis [87]. The cultured BMMNCs secreted 281.2 ± 85.0 pg of VEGF per 10^5 cells per day. Incorporation into the endothelial lining and production of angiogenic factors was thought to contribute to the protective effects against glomerular injury.

Table 3. Efficacy of EPCs or EPC product (EVs) on CKD in animal models

Author and Year	Animal	Model	Cell Type	Efficacy
Rookmaaker MB (2003)	Rat	Anti Thy1.1 GN	Rat Allogeneic BM Cell	Yes
Uchimura H (2005)	Rat	Anti Thy1.1 GN	Rat BMEPC	Yes
Sangidorj O (2010)	Mouse	5/6 Nephrectomy	Mouse Bmepc	Yes
Zhang Y (2012)	Mouse	Db/Db Type 2 Dm	Mouse Bmepc	Yes
Yuen DA (2013)	Rat	5/6 Nephrectomy	Rat BMEPC	Yes
Zhu XY (2013)	Pig	Renal Artery Stenosis	Pig PBEPC	Yes
Eirin A (2013)	Pig	Renal Artery Stenosis	Pig PBEPC	Yes
Cantaluppi V (2015)	Rat	Anti Thy1.1 GN	Human PBEPC-EV	Yes
Huang (2015)	Rat	5/6 Nephrectomy	Rat PBEPC	Yes

Subtotal nephrectomy (5/6 nephrectomy) model, a model of chronic renal failure by volume reduction of renal mass, was used in some articles for testing the efficacy of cell-based therapy on renal failure [88, 90, 94]. 5/6 nephrectomy model is suitable for CKD and renal fibrosis research because the condition is a good simulation of renal failure after loss of kidney function in humans [96, 97]. Sangidorj et al. provided externally administered allogeneic mouse BMEPCs significantly reduced deterioration of renal function, proteinuria, glomerular sclerosis, and interstitial fibrosis compared with 5/6 nephrectomized control animals [88]. Transplanted EPCs were present in glomerular capillaries and peritubular capillaries up to 8 weeks after the transfer. The renal expression of proinflammatory cytokines (IL-1β, TNF-α, IL-6) and adhesion molecules (MCP-1, ICAM-1, VCAM-1) was decreased in the EPC treated group at the early stage of disease. Inversely, the angiogenic molecules, including VEGF and KDR were restored by EPC treatment. Therefore, the EPC treatment switched the proinflammatory micro-environment of injured kidneys to the anti-inflammatory condition. Yuen et al. demonstrated BM-derived culture-modified cells (under endothelial cell culture), not stromal cells, significantly improved glomerulosclerosis and renal fibrosis compared with control animals (90). They also provided that, despite substantial improvement in the structure and function, BM-derived culture-modified cells were very rare in the kidney, suggesting that the effects are mediated by the secretion of diffusible anti-fibrotic factors. Huang et al. also confirmed the beneficial effects of EPCs on 5/6 nephrectomy rats [94]. They determined that kidney blood flow, serum creatinine levels, and the kidney injury score significantly improved by allogeneic rat PBEPC administration. Protein expression of apoptotic (caspase 3, PARP), inflammatory (TNF-α, MMP-9), oxidative stress (oxidized protein, NOX-1), fibrotic (Smad3, TGF-β), and hypoxic/ischemic cell-stress (HIF-1, p-Akt) biomarkers in the renal parenchyma all showed significant reduction compared with 5/6 nephrectomized control rats. On the other hand, angiogenesis at the protein (eNOS, CD31) and cellular ($CD31^+$, $CXCR4^+$) levels showed a parallel improvement with the improvement of blood flow. These results support that EPC therapy effectively inhibited the propagation of CKD and the deterioration of the renal function through the enhancement of angiogenesis, blood flow, and anti-oxidative capacity, as well as the suppression of inflammation, oxidative stress, apoptosis, and fibrosis in the animal model of CKD.

Zhang et al. provided the efficacy of EPCs on db/db mice, a model of type 2 diabetic nephropathy [89]. Exogenously administered cells, both diabetic and non-diabetic allogeneic early-outgrowth cells, equally ameliorated kidney injury (mesangial expansion, peritubular matrix expansion) and oxidative stress. They presumed that similar beneficial effects of cells from healthy and diabetic donors might highlight the potential of autologous cell therapy in a related clinical setting. Eirin et al. investigated the effect of EPCs on the swine model of renal artery stenosis [92]. The intrarenal delivery of autologous PB-derived endothelial outgrowth cells significantly increased the GFR, blood flow, and angiogenesis of stenotic kidney, and significantly attenuated the fibrosis. The endothelial outgrowth cells increased the cell proliferation and decreased the ratio of M1/M2 macrophages. Cultured endothelial outgrowth cells also released microvesicles *in vitro* and induced a phenotypic switch (M1 to M2) in cultured monocytes.

Recent advances in regenerative cell therapy indicates extracellular microvesicles (EVs) as important regulatory mediators for intercellular communication (main mechanism of paracrine action). The EVs were previously believed as "cell debris" in the circulation with unknown function. The horizontal transfer of several cargos containing cytokines, growth factor, and genetic information (DNA, mRNA, miRNA) from regeneration associated cells to target cells in the damaged organ promotes the tissue repairing process. External EVs administration has been challenged as to whether EVs restore organ damage as well as cell administration. Cantaluppi et al. examined the effect of EPCs-derived EVs on anti-Thy1.1 glomerulonephritis, complement and cytokine mediated glomerular injury [93]. EVs isolated from human EPCs, when injected intravenously, localized within injured glomeruli, and inhibited mesangial cell activation, leucocyte infiltration and adhesion, apoptosis, and ameliorated renal function. RNase pre-treatment of EVs abrogated their protective effects, suggesting the crucial role of RNA transfer from EVs to damaged glomerular cells. These EV-based cell-free biological therapy might be more biocompatible and less immunologic compared to a cell-based therapy. However, in cell-free EVs treatment, the repeated multiple administrations of programmed molecules or genetic materials might be necessary. In EPC-based cell therapy, EPCs, once administered, could synthesize and continuously secrete EVs without interruption, and subsequently could continuously carry EVs to target cells.

We recently found the efficacy of human UCB-derived QQc-cultured CD34+ EPCs in adenine-induced chronic tubulointerstitial injury in NOD/SCID mice (unpublished data). The metabolic product of adenine, 2,8-dihydroxyadenine (DHA), accumulates in the tubules and interstitium, and causes progressive tubular epithelial degeneration and interstitial fibrosis. The repeated administration of QQc-cultured CD34+ cells significantly improved the course of progressive kidney dysfunction, and restored histological damages, including tubular dilatation with tubular epithelial cell degeneration, and interstitial fibrosis. The effect of cell therapy was accompanied by better preservation of CD31+ PTCs (Figure 4). As is shown in AKI, the restoration of PTCs network is a critical factor for the inhibition of CKD progression.

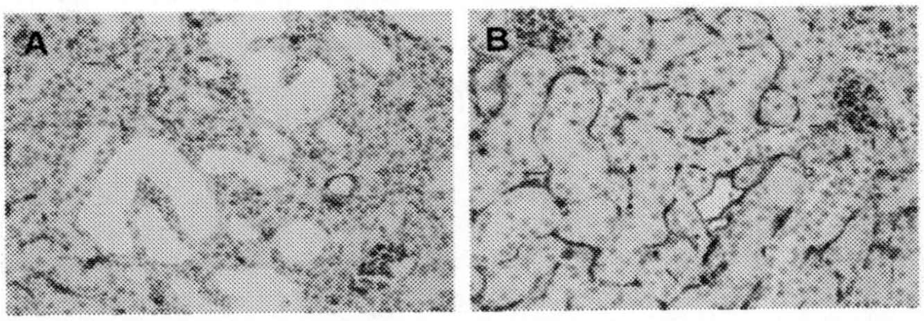

Figure 4. EPCs improve microvasculature loss in adenine-induced tubulointerstitial nephritis in mouse. (A) Adenine-induced chronic tubuointerstitial nephritis in NOD/SCID mice. PTCs located near degenerated and dilated tubules shows severe loss by CD31 immunostaining. (B) Repeated administration of human umbilical cord blood-derived $CD34^{+}$ EPCs significantly improved PTC loss and interstitial fibrosis. *Abbreviations: NOD-SCID = non-obese diabetic/severe combined immunodeficiency; PTC = peritubular capillary; EPC = endothelial progenitor cell.* (Unpublished data from author's institution).

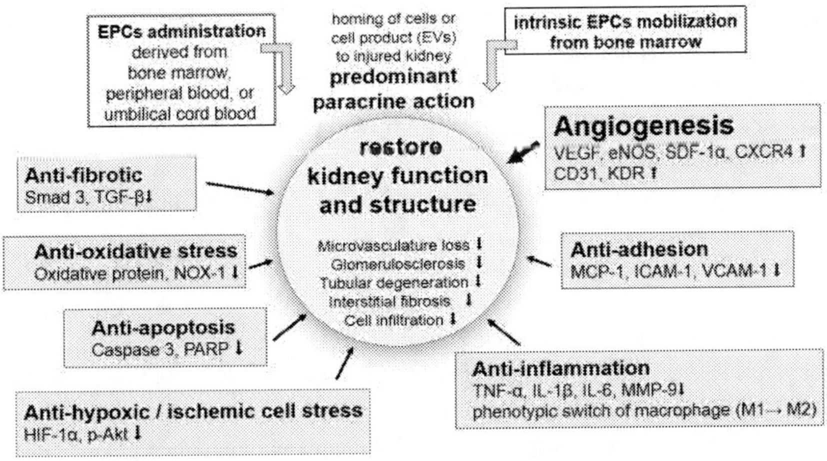

Figure 5. Mechanisms of therapeutic effects of EPC on kidney disease. Exogenously administered (or intrinsically mobilized) EPCs mainly act by paracrine mechanism to restore kidney injury. EPCs (or EVs secreted from EPCs) have a variety of actions beneficial to tissue repair including angiogenesis, anti-inflammatory, anti-adhesion, anti-hypoxic/ischemic cell stress, anti-apoptosis, anti-oxidative stress, and anti-fibrotic actions. Administration of EVs without donor EPCs (cell-free biological therapy) improved kidney injury in preclinical study. This protective effect of EVs is abrogated by RNase pretreatment of EVs, suggesting the crucial role of RNA transfer from EVs to damaged renal cells. Abbreviation: EPC = endothelial progenitor cells; EVs = extracellular vesicles.

As mentioned above, EPCs or its product EVs significantly induces tissue repair of chronic kidney damage. The proposed mechanisms underlying the positive therapeutic effects of EPCs on CKD are summarized in Figure 5.

EPC Therapy for Kidney Disease

Clinical Applications

AKI

AKI occurs in approximately 10-15% of patients admitted to the hospital, while its incidence in the intensive care unit has been reported in more than 50% of the patients [98-100]. In patients with severe AKI, a renal replacement therapy is performed to remove uremic substances, excessive water, and to correct electrolytes and acid-base abnormality. Acute uremic milieu induces a variety of disorders, including cardiac, respiratory, metabolic, and immune-ological dysfunctions, leading to increase in-hospital mortality [98-100]. The transition from AKI to CKD is also an important problem [100]. Even though the recovery from AKI is acquired, long-term damage in the kidney persists, and AKI-CKD transition further threatens the lives of patients. Although poor prognoses of AKI have already been well known, there has been no established effective treatment for human AKI.

There has been no clinical report in which $CD34^+$ cell therapy was applied to multiple patients with severe AKI. We started clinical research of G-CSF-mobilized autologous PB-derived $CD34^+$ cell transplantation for severe AKI as phase I clinical research and are now evaluating the safety and efficacy of the treatment. First-in-human case, in whom hemodialysis treatment was necessary for 2 weeks after admission, treated with $CD34^+$ cell therapy in our hospital showed no adverse events other than transient fever and thrombocytosis, and was observed to effectively recover from severe AKI [101]. The estimated GFR (eGFR) improved from 0.11 mL/min/1.73 m^2/day at pre-transplantation to 0.25 mL/min/1.73 m^2/day after cell therapy. Although careful monitoring and judgment about the safety and efficacy should be performed, a cell-based therapy using $CD34^+$ EPCs might be a promising optional treatment for severe AKI.

CKD

The first clinical trial of $CD34^+$ EPCs on CKD was reported by Lee et al. [102]. This phase I clinical trial was performed as followings: subjects; 10 patients with CKD at stage III or IV (eGFR 15~45 mL/min/1.73 m^2), cell source; granulocyte colony-stimulating factor-mobilized PB-derived autologous 5×10^7 $CD34^+$ cells, administration route; intra-renal arterial infusion into right renal artery, follow up; 12 months for evaluating the safety and efficacy of cell therapy. The procedure of intra-renal arterial infusion was safe in all the patients without adverse events. Serum creatinine maintained the same level between the baseline and at the end of one-year follow-up in the cell-treated group. Compared with the control group who failed to enroll into the trial at the initial state of eligibility assessment, cell-treated group did not show any beneficial effects [102].

Subsequently, the authors performed a randomized, open-label, controlled trial of autologous G-CSF mobilized $CD34^+$ cell transplantation in patients with CKD as a first phase II clinical trial to address the therapeutic efficacy [103]. CKD patients (stage III or IV) were randomly allocated into a treatment group (2.5×10^7 cells for each intrarenal artery; $n = 26$) and control group (standard pharmacotherapy; $n = 26$). The primary endpoint was safety and change of creatinine level/creatinine clearance; additionally, the secondary endpoints included 12-month combined unfavorable outcomes (death or dialysis), improvement of proteinuria, and $CD34^+$ cell-related adverse events. All the patients were uneventfully discharged after $CD34^+$ cell therapy. The one-year combined unfavorable clinical outcomes were significantly lower in the treatment group than in the control group ($p = 0.038$). However, the serum creatinine levels, ratio of urinary protein to urinary creatinine, and creatinine clearance showed no difference between the treatment group and control group ($p > 0.1$). The authors supposed potential extrarenal benefits of intrarenal artery infusion of autologous $CD34^+$ cells in the setting of advanced kidney disease.

Conclusion

Cell therapy using EPCs for AKI and CKD in humans is now underway and the challenges are continuing. Preclinical studies demonstrated a lot of promising benefits of EPC-based cell therapy in kidney disease. There still remains several issues to be verified, i.e. cell source, cell number, treatment frequency, autologous or allogeneic with some modulation, approach to enhance cell potential, and subjects to be treated. Cell-based therapy has been previously provided and evolved as an additional adjunctive therapy for no-optional patients with refractory disease. However, more common but clinically important disease such as kidney disease, due to which many patients suffer in the world, might be targeted, and cell therapy might be stated as one of the mainstream therapeutic strategies. Several patients with kidney disease might be able to receive benefits from cell-based therapy in the future.

References

[1] Ma L. J. Nakamura S. Whitsitt J. D. Davidson J. M. Fogo A. B. (2000). Regression of sclerosis in aging by an angiotensin inhibition-induced decrease in PAI-1. *Kidney Int* 58, 2425-36.

[2] Remuzzi A. Gagliardini E. Donadoni C. Fassi A. Sangalli F. (2002). Effect of angiotensin antagonism on the regression of kidney disase in the rat. *Kidney Int* 62, 885-94.

[3] Aldigier J. C. Kanjanbuch T. Ma L. J. Brown N. J. Fogo A. B. (2005). Regression of existing glomerulosclerosis by inhibition of aldosterone. *J Am Soc Nephrol* 16, 3306-14.

[4] Fiorreto P. Steffes M. W. Sutherland D. E. Goetz F. C. Mauer M. (1998). Reversal of lesions of diabetic nephropathy after pancreas transplantation. *N Engl J Med* 339, 69-75.

[5] Ohtake T. Oka M. Maesato K. Mano T. Ikee R. Moriya H. Kobayashi S. (2008). Pathological regression by angiotensin II type 1 receptor blockade in patients with mesangial proliferative glomerulonephritis. *Hypertens Res* 31, 387-94.

[6] Frazer S. D. S. Roderick P. J. (2019). Kidney disease in the global burden of disease study 2017. *Nat. Rev. Nephrol* 15, 193-4.

[7] Risdon R. A. Sloper J. C. De Wardener H.E. (1968). Relationship between renal function and histological changes found in renal-biopsy specimens from patients with persistent glomerular nephritis. *Lancet* 2, 363-6.

[8] Fine L. G. Bandyopadhay D. Norman J. T. (2000). Is there a common mechanism for the progression of different types of renal diseases other than proteinuria? Towards the unifying theme of chronic hypoxia. *Kidney Int* 75, S22-6.

[9] Nangaku M. (2006). Chronic hypoxia and tubulointerstitial injury: a final common pathway to end-stage renal failure. *J Am Soc Nephrol* 17: 17-25.

[10] Kang D. H. Kanellis J. Hugo C. Truong L. Anderson S. Kerjaschki D. Schreiner G. F. Johnson R. J. (2002). Role of microvascular endothelium in progressive renal disease. *J Am Soc Nephrol* 13, 806-16.

[11] Fine L. G. Orphanides C. Norman J. T. (1998). Progressive renal disease: the chronic hypoxia hypothesis. *Kidney Int* 65, S74-8.

[12] Norman J. T. Clark I. M. Garcia P. L. (2000). Hypoxia promotes fibrogenesis in human renal fibroblasts. *Kidney Int* 58, 2351-66.

[13] Bohre A. Mackensen-Haen S. Wehrmann M. (1996). Significance of post-glomerular capillaries in the pathogenesis of chronic renal failure. *Blood Press Res* 19, 191-5.

[14] Kobayashi S. Venkatachalam M. A. (1992). Differential effects of calorie restriction on glomeruli and tubules of the remnant kidney. *Kidney Int* 42, 710-7.

[15] Brezis M. Heyman S. N. Dinour D. Epstein F. H. Rosen S. (1991). Role of nitric oxide in renal medullary oxygenation. Studies in isolated and intact rat kidneys. *J Clin Invest* 88, 390-5.

[16] Schurek H. J. Jost U. Baumgartl H. Heckmann U. (1990). Evidence for a preglomerular oxygen diffusion shunt in rat renal cortex. *Am J Physiol* 259, F910-5.

[17] Welch W. J. Baumgartl H. Lubbers D. Wilcox C. S. (2001). Nephron pO_2 and oxygen usage in the hypertensive rat kidney. *Kidney Int 2001* 59, 230-7.

[18] Kobayashi S. Clemmons D. R. Nogami H. Roy A. K. Venkatachalam M. A. (1995). Tubular hypertrophy due to work load induced by furosemide is associated with increases of IGF-1 and IGFBP-1. *Kidney Int* 47, 818-28.

[19] Olof P. Hellberg A. Kallskog O. Wolgast M. (1991). Red cell trapping and postischemic renal blood flow. Differences between the cortex, outer and inner medulla. *Kidney Int* 40, 625-31.

[20] Vetterlein F. Petho A. Schmidt G. (1986). Distribution of capillary blood flow in rat kidney during postichemic renal failure. *Am J Physiol* 251, H510-9.

[21] Regner K. R. Zuk A. van Why S. K. Shames B. D. Ryan R. P. Falck J. R. Manthati V. L. McMullen M. E. Ledbetter S. R. Roman R. J. (2009). Protective effect of 20-HETE analogues in experimental renal ischemia reperfusion injury. *Kidney Int* 75, 511-7.

[22] Regner K. R. Roman R. J. (2012). Role of medullary blood flow in the pathogenesis of renal ischemia-reperfusion injury. *Curr Opin Nephrol Hypertens* 21, 33-38.

[23] Venkatachalam M. A. Weinberg J. M. Kriz W. Bidani A. K. (2015). Failed tubule recovery, AKI-CKD transition, and kidney disease progression. *J Am Soc Nephrol* 26, 1765-76.

[24] Basile D. P. Donohoe D. Roethe K. Osborn J. L. (2001). Renal ischemic injury results in permanent damage to peritubular capillaries and influences long-term function. *Am J Physiol Renal Physiol* 281, F887-99.

[25] Bunn H. F. (2013). Erythropoietin. *Cold Spring Harb Perspect Med* 3: a011619.

[26] Eckardt K. U. Koury S. T. Tan C. C. Schuster S. J. Kaissling B. Ratcliffe P. J. Kurtz A. (1993). Distribution of erythropoietin producing cells in rat kidneys during hypoxic hypoxia. *Kidney Int* 43, 815-23.

[27] Obara N. Suzuki N. Kim K. Nagasawa T. Imagawa S. Yamamoto M. (2008). Repression via the GATA box is essential for tissue-specific erythropoietin gene expression. *Blood* 111, 5223-32.

[28] Pan X. Suzuki N. Hirano I. Yamazaki S. Minegishi N. Yamamoto M. (2011). Isolation and characterization of renal erythropoietin-producing cells from genetically produced anemia mice. *PLoS One* 6, e25839.

[29] Souma T. Nezu M. Nakano D. Yamazaki S. Hirano I. Sekine H. Dan T. Takeda K. Fong GH. Nishiyama A. Ito S. Miyata T. Yamamoto M. Suzuki S. (2016). Erythropoietin synthesis in renal myofibroblast is restored by activation of hypoxia signaling. *J Am Soc Nephrol* 27, 428-38.

[30] Asada N. Takase M. Namakura J. Oguchi A. Asada M. Suzuki N. Yamamura K. Nagoshi N. Shibata S. Rao T. N. Fehling H. J. Fukatsu A. Minegishi N. Kita T.

Kimura T. Okano H. Yamamoto M. Yanagita M. (2011). Dysfunction of fibroblast of extrarenal origin underlies renal fibrosis and renal anemia in mice. *J Clin Invest* 121, 3981-90.

[31] Griendling K. K. Minieri C. A. Ollerenshaw J. D. Alexander R. W. (1994). Angiotensin II stimulates NADH and NADPH oxidase activity in cultured vascular smooth muscle cells. *Circ Res* 74, 1141-8.

[32] Johnson R. J. Alpers C. E. Yoshimura A. Lombardi D. Pritzl P. Floege J. Schwartz S. M. (1992). Renal injury from angiotensin II-mediated hypertension. *Hypertension* 19, 464-74.

[33] Kobayashi S. Ishida A. Moriya H. Mori N. Fukuda T. Takamura T. (1999). Angiotensin II receptor blockade limits kidney injury in two-kidney, one-clip Goldblatt hypertensive rats with special reference to phenotypic changes. *J Lab Clin Med* 133, 134-43.

[34] Kobayashi S. Moriya H. Nakabayashi I. Nishiyama J. Fukuda T. (2002). Angiotensin II and IGF-1 may interact to regulate tubulointerstitial cell kinetics and phenotypic changes in hypertensive rats. *Hypertens Res* 25, 257-69.

[35] Ferrara N. (1999). Role of vascular endothelial growth factor in the regulation of angiogenesis. *Kidney Int* 56, 794-814.

[36] Brown L. F. Berse B. Tognazzi K. Manseau E. J. Van de Water L. Senger D. R. Dvorak H. F. Rosen S. (1992). Vascular permeability factor mRNA and protein expression in human kidney. *Kidney Int* 42, 1457-61.

[37] Kang D. H. Anderson S. Kim Y. G. Mazzalli M. Suga S. Jefferson J. A. Gordon K. L. Oyama T. T. Hughes J. Hugo C. Kerjaschki D. Schreiner G. F. Johnson R. J. (2001). Impaired angiogenesis in the aging kidney: vascular endothelial growth factor and thrombospondin-1 in renal disease. *Am J Kidney Dis* 37, 601-11.

[38] Kong T. Eltzschig H. K. Karhausen J. Colgan S. P. Shelley C. S. (2004). Leukocyte adhesion during hypoxia is mediated by HIF-1-dependent induction of beta 2 integrin gene expression. *Pro Natl Acad Sci USA* 101, 10440.

[39] Masuda Y. Shimizu A. Mori T. Ishiwata T. Kitamura H. Ohashi R. Ishizaki M. Asano G. Sugisaki Y. Yamanaka M. (2001). Vascular endothelial growth factor enhances glomerular capillary repair and accelerates resolution of experimentally induced glomerulonephritis. *Am J Pathol* 159, 599-608.

[40] Kang D. H. Hughes J. Mazzali M. Schreiner G. F. Johnson R. J. (2001). Impaired angiogenesis in the remnant kidney model: II. Vascular endothelial growth factor administration reduces renal fibrosis and stabilizes renal function. *J Am Soc Nephrol* 12, 1448-57.

[41] Go A. S. Chertow G. M. Fan D. McCulloh C. E. Hsu C. Y. (2004). Chronic kidney disease and the risk of death, cardiovascular events, and hospitalization. *N Engl J Med* 351, 1296-305.

[42] Herzog C. A. Asinger R. W. Berger A. K. Charytan D. M. Diez J. Hart R. G. Eckardt K. U. Kasiske B. L. McCullough P. A. Passman R. S. Deloach S. S. Pun P. H. Ritz E. (2011). Cardiovascular disease in chronic kidney disease. A clinical update from kidney disease: Improving Global Outcomes (KDIGO). *Kidney Int* 80, 572-86.

[43] Ohtake T. Kobayashi S. Moriya H. Negishi K. Okamoto K. Maesato K. Saito S. (2005). High prevalence of occult coronary artery stenosis in patients with chronic kidney disease at the initiation of renal replacement therapy: an angiographic examination. *J Am Soc Nephrol* 16, 1141-8.

[44] Kobayashi S. Ikeda T. Moriya H. Ohtake T. Kumagai H. (2004). Asymptomatic cerebral lacunae in patients with chronic kidney disease. *Am J Kidney Dis* 44, 35-41.

[45] Sarnak M. J. Levey A. S. (2000). Cardiovascular disease and chronic kidney disease: a new paradigm. *Am J Kidney Dis* 35 (Suppl 1): S117-31.

[46] Drew D. A. Sarnak M. J. (2014). Ischemic and hemorrhagic stroke: high incidence in hemodialysis and peritoneal dialysis patients. *Am J Kidney Dis* 63, 547-8.

[47] Jourde-Chiche N. Dou L. Cerini C. Dignat-George F. Brunet P. (2011). Vascular incompetence in dialysis patients–protein-bound uremic toxins and endothelial dysfunction. *Seminar Dial* 24, 327-37.

[48] Stam F. van Guldener C. Becker A. Dekker J. M. Heine R. J. Bouter L. M. Stehouwer C. D. A. (2006). Endothelial dysfunction contributes to renal function-associated cardiovascular mortality in a population of mild renal insufficiency: The Hoorn Study. *J Am Soc Nephrol* 17, 537-45.

[49] Ohtake T. Ishioka K. Honda K. Oka M. Maesato K. Mano T. Ikee R. Moriya H. Hidaka S. Kobayashi S. (2010). Impact of coronary artery calcification in hemodialysis patients: risk factors and associations with prognosis. *Hemodial Int* 14, 218-25.

[50] Ohtake T. Oka M. Ikee R. Mochida Y. Ishioka K. Moriya H. Hidaka S. Kobayashi S. (2011). Impact of lower limbs' arterial calcification on the prevalence and severity of PAD in patients on hemodialysis. *J Vasc Surg* 53, 676-83.

[51] Kobayashi S. (2016). Cardiovascular events in chronic kidney disease (CKD) -an importance of vascular calcification and microcirculatory impairment. *Renal Replacement Therapy* 2, 55.

[52] Ohtake T. Kobayashi S. (2017). Impact of vascular calcification on cardiovascular mortality in hemodialysis patients: clinical significance, mechanisms, and possible strategies for treatment. *Renal Replacement Therapy* 3, 13.

[53] Annuk M. Zilmer M. Lind L. Linde T. Fellstrom B. (2001). Oxidative stress and endothelial function in chronic renal failure. *J Am Soc Nephrol* 12, 2747-52.

[54] Vasa M. Fichtlschere S. Aicher A. Urbich C. Martin H. Zeiher A. M. Dimmeler S. (2001). Number and migratory activity of circulating endothelial progenitor cells inversely correlate with risk factors for coronary artery disease. *Circ Res* 89, E1-7.

[55] de Groot K. Bahlmann F. H. Sowa J. Koenig J. Menne J. Haller H. Fliser D. (2004). Uremia causes endothelial progenitor cell deficiency. *Kidney Int* 66, 641-6.

[56] Krenning G. Dankers P. Y. W. Drouven J. W. Waanders F. Franssen C. F. M, van Luyn M. J. A. Harmsen M. C. Popa E. R. (2009). Endothelial progenitor cell dysfunction in patients with progressive kidney disease. *Am J Physiol Renal Physiol* 296, F1314-22.

[57] Jie K. E. Zaikova M. A. Bergevoet M. W. T. Westerweel P. E. Rastmanesh M. Blankestijn P. J. Boer W. H. Braam B. VerHaar M. C. (2010). Progenitor cells and

vascular function are impaired in patients with chronic kidney disease. *Nephrol Dial Transplant* 25, 1875-82.

[58] Choi J. H. Kim K. L. Huh W. Kim B. Byun J. Suh W. Sung J. Jeon E. S. Oh H. Y. Kim D. K. (2004). Decreased number and impaired angiogenic function of endothelial progenitor cells in patients with chronic renal failure. *Arterioscler Thromb Vasc Biol* 24, 1246-52.

[59] Eizawa T. Murakami Y. Matsui K. Takahashi M. Muroi K. Amemiya M. Takano R. Kusano E. Shimada K. Ikeda U. (2003). Circulating endothelial progenitor cells are reduced in hemodialysis patients. *Curr Med Res Opin* 19, 627-33.

[60] Schlieper G. Hristov M. Brandenburg V. Kruger T. Westenfeld R. Mahnken A. H. Yagmur E. Boeker G. Heussen N. Gladziwa U. Ketteler M. Weber C. Floege J. (2008). Predictors of low circulating endothelial progenitor cell number in haemodialysis patients. *Nephrol Dial Transplant* 23: 2611-8.

[61] Westerweel P. E. Peter I. E. H. Blankestijn P. J. de Bree P. Groeneveld D. van Oostrom O. Braam B. Koomans H. A. Verhaar M. C. (2007). End-stage renal disease causes an imbalance between endothelial and smooth muscle progenitor cells. *Am J Physiol Renal Physiol* 292, F1132-40.

[62] D'Apolito M. Colia A. L. Lasalvia M. Capozzi V. Falcone M. P. Pettoello-Mantovani M. Brownlee M. Maffione A. B. Giardino I. (2017). Urea-induced ROS accelerate senescence in endothelial progenitor cells. *Atherosclerosis* 263, 127-36.

[63] Maruyama S. Taguchi A. Iwashima S. Ozaki T. Yasuda K. Kikuchi-Taura A. Soma T. Ishii H. Murohara T. Takahashi H. Kasuga H. Kumada Y. Toriyama T. Ito Y. Kawahara H. Yuzawa Y. Matsuo S. (2008). Low circulating $CD34^+$ cell count is associated with poor prognosis in chronic hemodialysis patients. *Kidney Int* 74, 1603-9.

[64] Gremmels H. van Rhijn-Brouwer F. C. C. Papazova D. A. Fledderus J. O. Teraa M. Verhaar M. C. JUVENTAS Study group. (2019). Exhaustion of the bone marrow progenitor cell reserve is associated with major events in severe limb ischemia. *Angiogenesis* 22, 411-20.

[65] Naito T. Sanaka T. Mikami H. Soga A. Yamatani K. Segawa K. Kawashima M. Yoshikura T. Niwayama J. Nishimura H. Ogawa T. Ando A. Teramoto A. Nitta K. (2016). Modulation of circulating endothelial progenitor cells by erythropoiesis-stimulating agents in patients with chronic kidney disease stage G5 and 5D. *Clin Nephrol* 86, 242-52.

[66] Mohler 3rd E. R. Zhang L. Medenilla E. Rogers W. French B. Bantly A. Moore J. S. Huan Y. Murashima M. Berns J. (2011). Effect of darbepoietin alfa on endothelial progenitor cells and vascular reactivity in chronic kidney disease. *Vasc Med* 16, 183-9.

[67] Aicher A. Heeschen C. Mildner-Rihm C. Ulbich C. Ihling C. Technau-Ihling K. Zeiher A. M. Dimmeler S. (2003). Essential role of endothelial nitric oxide synthase for mobilization of stem and progenitor cells. *Nat Med* 9, 1370-6.

[68] Kobayashi S. Oka M. Maesato K. Ikee R. Mano T. Moriya H. Ohtake T. (2008). Coronary artery calcification, ADMA, and insulin resistance in CKD patients. *Clin J Am Soc Nephrol* 3, 1289-95.

[69] Fujii H. Li S. H. Szmitko P. E. Fedak P. W. M. Verma S. (2006). C-reactive protein alters antioxidant defenses and promotes apoptosis in endothelial progenitor cells. *Arterioscler Thromb Vasc Biol* 26. 2476-82.

[70] Verma S. Kuliszewski M. A. Li S. H. Szmitko P. E. Zuco L. Wang C. H. Badiwala M. V. Mickle D. A. G. Weisel R. D. Fedak P. W. M. Stewart D. J. Kutryk M. J. B. (2004). C-reactive protein attenuates endothelial progenitor cell survival, differentiation, and function: further evidence of a mechanistic link between C-reactive protein and cardiovascular disease. *Circulation* 109, 2058-67.

[71] Imanishi T. Hano T. Sawamura T. Nishio I. (2004). Oxidized low density-lipoprotein induces endothelial progenitor cell senescence, leading to cellular dysfunction. *Clin Exp Pharmacol Physiol* 31, 407-13.

[72] Imanishi T. Hano T. Nishio I. (2005). Angiotensin II accelerates endothelial progenitor cell senescence through induction of oxidative stress. *J Hypertens* 23, 97-104.

[73] Wu V. C. Young G. H. Huang P. H. Lo S. C. Wang K. C. Sun C. Y. Liang C. J. Huang T. M. Chen J. H. Chang F. C. Chen Y. L. Kuo Y. S. Chen J. B. Chen J. W. Chen Y. M. Ko W. J. Wu K. D. NSARF group. (2013). In acute kidney injury, indoxyl sulfate impairs human endothelial progenitor cells: modulation by statin. *Angiogenesis* 16, 609-24.

[74] Barreto F. C. Barreto D. V. Liabeuf S. Meert N. Glorieux G. Temmar M. Choukroun G. Vanholder R. Massy Z. A. European Uremic Toxin Work Group (EU Tox). (2009). Serum indoxyl sulfate is associated with vascular disease and mortality in chronic kidney disease patients. *Clin J Am Soc Nephrol* 4, 1551-8.

[75] Ohtake T. Mochida Y. Ishioka K. Moriya H. Hidaka S. Hirata M. Yamada H. Kumagai H. Kobayashi S. (2020). Improvement of microcirculatory impairment in patients with predialysis chronic kidney disease after AST-120 administration. *Renal Replacement Therapy* 6, 28.

[76] Hung S. C. Kuo K. L. Huang H. L. Lin C. C. Tsai T. H. Wang C. H. Chen J. W. Lin S. J. Huang P. H. Tarng D. C. (2016). Indoxyl sulfate suppresses endothelial progenitor cell-mediated neovascularization. *Kidney Int* 89, 574-85.

[77] Hohenstein B. Kuo M.C. Addabbo F. Yasuda K. Ratliff B. Schwarzenberger C. Eckardt K. U. Hugo C. P. M. Goligorsky M. S. (2010). Enhanced progenitor cell recruitment and endothelial repair after selective endothelial injury of the mouse kidney. *Am J Physiol Renal Physiol* 298, F1504-14.

[78] Patschan D. Krupincza K. Patschan S. Zhang Z. Hamby C. Goligorsky M. S. (2006). Dynamics of mobilization and homing of endothelial progenitor cells after acute renal ischemia: modulation by ischemic preconditioning. *Am J Physiol Renal physiol* 291, F176-85.

[79] Dekel B. Shezen E. Even-Tov-Friedman S. Katchman H. Margalit R. Nagler A. Reisner Y. (2006). Transplantation of human hematopoietic stem cells into ischemic and growing kidneys suggest a role in vasculogenesis but not tubulogenesis. *Stem Cells Transl Med* 24, 1185-93.

[80] Li B. Cohen A. Hudson T. E. Motlagh D. Amrani D. L. Duffield J. S. (2010). Mobilized human hematopoietic stem/progenitor cells promote kidney repair after ischemia/reperfusion injury. *Circulation* 121, 2211-20.

[81] Cantaluppi V. Gatti S. Medica D. Figliolini F. Bruno S. Deregibus M. C. Sordi A. Biancone L. Tetta C. Camussi G. (2012). Microvesicles derived from endothelial progenitor cells protect the kidney from ischemia-reperfusion injury by mirco-RNA-dependent reprogramming of resident renal cells. *Kidney Int* 82, 412-27.

[82] Li L. Black R. Ma Z. Yang Q. Wang A. Lin F. (2012). Use of mouse hematopoietic stem and progenitor cells to treat acute kidney injury. *Am J Physiol Renal Physiol* 32, F9-19.

[83] Burger D. Vinas J. L. Akbari S. Dehak H. Knoll W. Gutsol A. Carter A. Touyz R. M. Allan D. S. Burns K. D. (2015). Human endothelial colony-forming cells protect against acute kidney injury. *Am J Pathol* 185, 2309-23.

[84] Ohtake T. Kobayashi S. Slavin S. Mochida Y. Ishioka K. Moriya H. Hidaka S. Matsuura R. Sumida M. Katagiri D. Noiri E. Okada K. Mizuno H. Tanaka R. (2018). Human peripheral blood mononuclear cells incubated in vasculogenic conditioning medium dramatically improve ischemia/reperfusion acute kidney injury in mice. *Cell Transplantation* 27, 520-30.

[85] Masuda H. Iwasaki H. Kawamoto A. Akimaru H. Ishikawa M. Ii M. Shizuno T. Sato A. Ito R. Horii M. Ishida H. Kato S. Asahara T. (2012). Development of serum-free quality and quantity control culture of colony-forming endothelial progenitozr cell for vasculogenesis. *Stem Cells Transl Med* 1, 160-71.

[86] Rookmaaker M. B. Smits A. M. Tolboom H. Van't Wout K. Martens A. C. Goldschmeding R. Joles J. A. Jan Van Zonneveld A. Grone H. J. Rabelink T. J. Verhaar M. C. (2003). Bone-marrow-derived cells contribute to glomerular endothelial repair in experimental glomerulonephritis. *Am J Pathol* 163, 553-62.

[87] Uchimura H. Marumo T. Takase O. Kawachi H. Shimizu F. Hayashi M. Saruta T. Hishikawa K. Fujita T. (2005). Intrarenal injection of bone marrow-derived angiogenic cells rescues endothelial injury and mesangial cell activation in experimental glomerulonephritis. *J Am Soc Nephrol* 16, 997-1004.

[88] Sangidorj O. Yang S. H. Jang H. R. Lee J. P. Cha RH, Kim S. M. Lim C. S. Kim Y. S. (2010). Bone marrow-derived endothelial progenitor cells confer renal protection in a murine chronic renal failure model. *Am J Pathol* 299: F325-35.

[89] Zhang Y. Yuen D. A. Advani A. Thai K. Advani S. L. Kepecs D. Kabir M. G. Connelly K. A. Gilbert R. E. (2012). Early-outgrowth bone marrow cells attenuate renal injury and dysfunction via an antioxidant effect in a mouse model of type 2 diabetes. *Diabetes* 61, 2114-25.

[90] Yuen D. A. Connelly K. A. Advani A. Liao C. Kuliszewski M. A. Trogadis J. Thai K. Advani S. L. Zhang Y. Kelly D. J. Leong-Poi H. Keating A. Marsden P. A. Stewart D. J. Gilbert R. E. (2010). Culture-modified bone marrow cells attenuate cardiac and renal injury in a chronic kidney disease rat model via a novel antifibrotic mechanism. *PLoS One* 5, e9543.

[91] Zhu X. Y. Urbieta-Caceres V. Krier J. D. Textor S. C. Lerman A. Lerman L. O. (2013). Mesenchymal stem cells and endothelial progenitor cells decrease renal injury in experimental swine renal artery stenosis though different mechanism. *Stem Cells* 31, 117-25.

[92] Eirin A. Zhu X. Y. Li Z. Ebrahimi B. Zhang X. Tang H. Korsmo M. J. Chade A. R. Grande J. P. Ward C. J. Simari R. D. Lerman A. Textor S. C. Lerman L. O.

(2013). Endothelial outgrowth cells shift macrophage phenotype and improve kidney viability in swine renal artery stenosis. *Arterioscler Thromb Vasc Biol* 33, 1006-13.

[93] Cantaluppi V. Medica D. Mannari C. Stiaccini G. Figliolini F. Dellepiane S. Quercia A. D. Migliori M. Panichi V. Giovannini L. Bruno S. Tetta C. Biancone L. Camussi G. (2015). Endothelial progenitor cell-derived extracellular vesicles protect from complement-mediated mesangial injury in experimental anti-Thy1.1 glomerulonephritis. *Nephrol Dial Transplant* 30, 410-22.

[94] Huang T. H. Chen Y. T. Sung P. H. Chiang H. J. Chen Y. L. Chai H. T. Chung S. Y. Tsai T. H. Yang C. C. Chen C. H. Chen Y. L. Chang H. W. Sun C. K. Yip H. K. (2015). Peripheral blood-derived endothelial progenitor cell therapy prevented deterioration of chronic kidney disease in rats. *Am J Transl Med* 7, 804-24.

[95] Kawachi H. Orikasa M. Matsui K. Iwanaga T. Toyabe S. Oite T. Shimizu F. (1992). Epitope-specific induction of mesangial lesion with proteinuria by a MoAB against mesangial cell surface antigen. *Clin Exp Immunol* 88, 399-404.

[96] Yang H. C. Zuo Y. Fogo A. B. (2010). Models of chronic kidney disease. *Drug Discov Today Dis Models* 7, 13-9.

[97] Lim B. J. Yang H. C. Fogo A. B. (2014). Animal models of regression/progression of kidney disease. *Drug Discov Today Dis Models* 11, 45-51.

[98] Ronco C. Bellomo R. Kellum J. A. (2019). Acute kidney injury. *Lancet* 394, 1949-64.

[99] Hoste E. A. Bagshaw S.M. Bellomo R. Cely C. M. Colman R. Cruz D. N. Edipidis K. Forni L. G. Gomersall C. D. Govil D. Honore P. M. Joannes-Boyau O. Joannidis M. Korhonen A.M. Lavrentieva A. Mehta R. L. Palevsky P. Roessler E. Ronco C. Uchino S. Vazquez J. A. Andrade E. V. Webb S. Kellum J. A. (2015). Epidemiology of acute kidney injury in critically ill patients: the multinational AKI-EPI study. *Intensive Care Med* 41, 1411-23.

[100] Chawla L. S. Eggers P. W. Star R. A. Kimmel P. L. (2014). Acute kidney injury and chronic kidney disease as interconnected syndromes. *N Engl J Med* 371, 58-66.

[101] Suzuki H. Ohtake T. Tsukiyama T. Morota M. Ishioka K. Moriya H. Mochida Y. Hidaka S. Sato T. Asahara T. Kobayahsi S. (2021). Acute kidney injury successfully treated with autologous granulocyte colony-stimulating factor-mobilized peripheral blood CD34-positive cell transplantation: A first-in-human report. *Stem Cells Transl Med* 10, 1253-7.

[102] Lee M. S. Lee F. Y. Chen Y. L. Sung P. H. Chiang H. J. Chen K. H. Huang T. H. Chen Y. L. Chiang J. Y. Yin T. C. Chang H. W. Yip H. K. (2017). Investigated the safety of intra-renal arterial transfusion of autologous CD34+ cells and time course of creatinine levels, endothelial dysfunction biomarkers and micro-RNAs in chronic kidney disease patients-phase I clinical trial. *Oncotarget* 8, 17750-62.

[103] Yang C. C. Sung P. H. Cheng B. C. Li Y. C. Chen Y. L. Lee M. S. Yip H. K. (2020). Safety and efficacy of intrarenal arterial autologous CD34+ cell transfusion in patients with chronic kidney disease: A randomized, open-label controlled phase II clinical trial. *Stem Cells Transl Med* 9, 827-38.

Section V: EPC Derived Extracellular Vesicles

Chapter 8

Therapeutic Applications of Endothelial Progenitor Cell-Derived Extracellular Vesicles in Cardiovascular Diseases

Junjie Yang[1,*] and Jiacheng Sun[2]

[1]Department of Anesthesiology,
University of Maryland School of Medicine,
Baltimore, Maryland, USA
[2]Department of Biomedical Engineering,
University of Alabama at Birmingham,
School of Medicine and School of Engineering,
Birmingham, Maryland, USA

Abstract

Despite the advances in the treatment of cardiovascular diseases (CVDs), CVDs remain the leading cause of global mortality and a major contributor to disability. Translational cell therapies using endothelial progenitor cells (EPCs) hold great promise due to their potential to secrete protective cytokines and their ability to differentiate into endothelial cells. In fact, several studies have attributed the therapeutic effects of transplanted EPCs to their strong secretory effect, namely extracellular vesicles (EVs), rather than the direct differentiation of adherent cells. Moreover, accumulating preclinical and clinical studies have proved the therapeutic effect of EPC-EVs, which carry various lipids, proteins, and microRNAs, in multiple cardiovascular diseases. Transplanted EPC-EVs have been shown to accumulate at injury sites of the heart or blood vessels, exerting various effects, including pro-

[*] Corresponding Author's Email: junjieyang2009@gmail.com.

In: Endothelial Progenitor Cells in Health and Disease
Editors: Amankeldi A. Salybekov, Shuzo Kobayashi and Takayuki Asahara
ISBN: 978-1-68507-794-5

angiogenesis, anti-inflammation, anti-oxidation, anti-apoptosis, anti-vascular remodeling, and the inhibition of endothelial-to-mesenchymal transition as well as cardiac fibrosis (Figure 1). In this chapter, we have summarized the findings from recent research on the biological functions and the potential therapeutic applications of EPC-EVs in cardiovascular diseases.

Keywords: endothelial progenitor cells, extracellular vesicles: cardiovascular diseases, angiogenesis, therapeutics

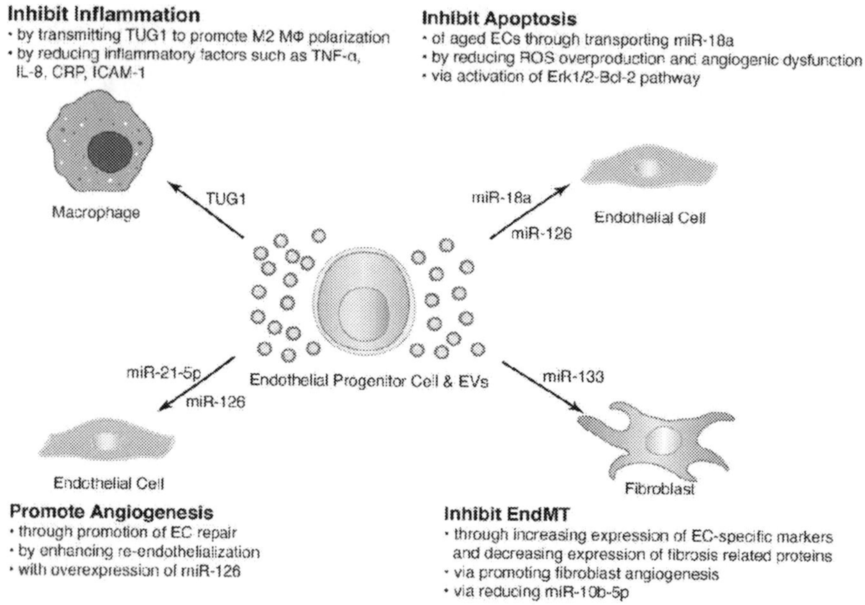

Figure 1. Effect of EPC-EVs to various cell types.

Introduction

Accounting for more than 17.9 million deaths a year, cardiovascular diseases (CVDs) remain the most common cause of death in the world. Despite significant advances in the medical treatment of CVDs, such as drug treatment, surgery, and interventional therapy, heart diseases remain a major cause of death and a long-term condition. Although traditional therapeutic strategies can improve symptoms and alleviate adverse cardiac remodeling, there is no available treatment aiming to reduce the irreversible loss of cardiomyocytes.

Stem cell therapy has been demonstrated to be a promising therapeutic approach for the treatment of CVDs due to their characteristics of self-renewal and multilineage-differentiation. Over the last two decades, several pre-clinical and clinical studies have revealed the great potential and safety of different types of stem cells, including mesenchymal stem cell (MSCs) [1-3], endothelial progenitor cells (EPCs) [4-7], embryonic stem cells (ESCs) [8], and induced pluripotent stem cells (iPSCs) [9]. Although several studies have demonstrated encouraging results with stem cells, there are still some drawbacks, such as poor retention and survival, tumorigenicity, and immune rejection limiting the development of these new strategies. In fact, the paracrine release of bioactive molecules is being accepted as the most acceptable mechanism to interpret the beneficial effects of cell therapy. Studies have confirmed that stem cell-derived extracellular vesicles (EVs) exert cardioprotective functions similar to stem cells, including the promotion of angiogenesis, decrease in apoptosis, and inhibition of fibrosis. Compared with stem cells, EVs have many desirable advantages, such as low toxicity, low immunogenicity, high stability in circulation, biocompatibility, and biological barrier permeability. Furthermore, EVs transport various active biomolecules from the heart to the recipient cells. Therefore, EVs stand for a promising therapy for CVDs, shifting the focus from stem cell therapy to cell-free, EV therapeutic approaches [10-12].

Extracellular Vesicles and Their Origin, Biogenesis, and Composition

Extracellular vesicles are generally categorized into three main subtypes, namely ectosomes, exosomes, and apoptotic bodies [13, 14], which are differentiated based upon their biogenesis, size, content, and function [15, 16]. Ectosomes, with a size of 50-1000 nm, also referred to as microvesicles, are formed by the direct outward budding of the cell's plasma membrane [17]. Apoptotic bodies are released by dying cells into the extracellular space, ranging in size from 50–5000 nm in diameter [18]. Unlike ectosomes and apoptotic bodies, exosomes, typically 30–150 nm in diameter, form by twice inward budding of membrane [17]. The first inward budding of the plasma membrane forms an early endosome, while the second inward budding of endosome membrane induces the formation of multivesicular bodies (MVB) that contain various intraluminal vesicles (ILVs) [14].

It is widely accepted that early endosomes mature in several ways to form late endosomes. They increase in size through homotypic fusion and increase in acidity through the activity of the V-ATPase [19, 20]. At the same time, small intraluminal vesicles (ILVs), charged with protein, lipids, nucleic acids or other cellular components, are formed by the budding of the endosome membrane into the endosome lumen, which leads to the multivesicular appearance of late endosomes, known as multivesicular bodies (MVBs) [21, 22]. MVBs and lysosomes rapidly exchange membrane components *in vivo*, forming a transient hybrid endo-lysosome. At this stage, the distinction between late endosomes, endo-lysosomes, and lysosomes is often obscure [23]. MVBs can also transport to the plasma membrane through cytoskeletal and microtubule network and fuse with the plasma membrane as secretory vesicles; the important content is found inside the MVBs exosome. The released exosomes, packaged with cellular molecules, can be distributed in the extracellular microenvironment, and upon delivery to target cells, regulate a wide range of cellular functions at a distance [24].

EVs can mediate intercellular communication that modulates the physiological state of the cells. Most of the EVs constitutively express certain molecules, including tetraspanins (CD9, CD63, CD81, and CD82), heat shock proteins (heat shock protein 70 and heat shock protein 90), Rab GTPases, flotillin, Alix, TSG101, regardless of the source [25, 26]. The contents of EVs from various types of cells are different; thus, they can exert different biological functions. It is reported that EVs can cargo a wide variety of molecules including proteins, lipids, DNAs, mRNAs, and miRNAs [27, 28]. Among these molecules, miRNAs are abundant and have attracted the most attention, due to their regulatory roles in gene expression. EVs derived from different cellular origins contain a unique expression profile of miRNAs, which may also differ from those of the parent cells [29]. MiRNAs in EVs may be utilized as important biomarkers for the early detection of several diseases, including CVDs, cancers, and diabetes [30-32]. Importantly, various studies have shown that miRNAs in EVs have a key regulatory role in CVDs [33-35].

Extracellular Vesicles Derived from Endothelial Progenitor Cells

Endothelial progenitor cells (EPCs) constitute one of the most broadly used stem cells for the treatment of CVDs. EPCs could differentiate into endothelial cells and incorporate into sites of neovascularization in the animal models of ischemia. For instance, systemically injected EPCs can be recruited into the ischemic myocardium and promote neovascularization and regeneration of ischemic tissues [36, 37]. The therapeutic effects of transplanted EPCs were attributed to the secretion of paracrine factors, including EVs [38, 39]. EPC-derived EVs are membrane vesicles 30–2000 nm in diameter that are secreted by EPCs under pathophysiological conditions. They have multiple functions in restoring cardiovascular dysfunction, such as anti-inflammation, anti-apoptosis, inhibition of cardiac fibrosis, and angiogenesis in CVDs. Except for common EV markers, EPC-EVs also carry markers with EPCs signatures, such as CD34, KDR, and VEGFR-2, and exhibited similar functions with EPCs, including enhancing EC proliferation and promoting angiogenesis [25]. Importantly, EPC-EVs have abundant levels of miRNAs, and are especially rich in proangiogenic and cardioprotective miRNAs, such as miR-133 and miR-486 [40, 41]. The release of EPC-EVs can be affected by external stimuli, such as inflammation, hypoxia, and exercise [42-44]. Thus, EVs derived from EPCs under different pathophysiological settings may have diverse intraluminal contents and functions.

Therapeutic Potential of EPC-derived EVs for Cardiovascular System

Anti-inflammation

Vascular inflammation and oxidative stress are the major triggers for CVDs. Chronic vascular inflammation leads to endothelial cell damage, atherosclerosis, vascular remodeling, and cardiovascular complications. Thus, the value of anti-inflammation therapy for the treatment of CVDs has been more and more recognized. EPC-derived EVs have been demonstrated to inhibit inflammatory reactions both *in vitro* and *in vivo* [45, 46]. Bai et al. demonstrated that treatment with EPC-derived EVs significantly reduced the production of inflammatory factors, including tumor TNF-α, IL-8, CRP, and

ICAM-1 in a mouse model of diabetes [47]. In hypoxia/reoxygenation (H/R) injury, treatment with ECFC-derived EVs blocked H/R-induced expression of the proinflammatory proteins, such as ICAM-1 and endothelial cell apoptosis [48]. Taurine upregulated gene 1 (TUG1), a long noncoding RNA (lncRNA), was downregulated in CLP-induced sepsis, and its re-expression can induce anti-inflammatory macrophage polarization and suppress macrophage-medicated inflammatory injury. Ma et al. reported that EPCs-derived EVs transmitted TUG1 to promote M2 macrophage polarization where TUG1 competitively bound to microRNA-9-5p (miR-9-5p) to upregulate the expression of sirtuin 1 (SIRT1) [49]. Therefore, the inhibition of inflammation is one of the prominent mechanisms of EPC-EVs' protective effects in CVDs.

Anti-Apoptosis

Myocardial apoptosis occurs in several CVDs, such as atherosclerosis, heart failure, ventricular remodeling, and peripheral arterial diseases. As a paracrine mechanism, stem cells-derived EVs take an active role in the inhibition of myocardial apoptosis [50, 51]. It was found that angiotensin-converting enzyme 2 (ACE2)-primed EPC-EVs could inhibit the apoptosis of aged endothelial cells after H/R injury through transporting miR-18a and subsequently down-regulating the Nox2/ROS pathway [52, 53]. In a separate study, Ma et al. reported that EPC-EVs protect ECs against H/R injury by reducing H/R-induced EC apoptosis, ROS overproduction, angiogenic dysfunction, and improving mitochondrial function [54]. Additionally, EPC-MVs with miR-126 overexpression reduced apoptosis of MC3T3-E1 cell via the activation of the Erk1/2-Bcl-2 pathway [55]. In summary, EPC-EVs are involved in the process of anti-apoptosis.

Inhibition of Cardiac Fibrosis

Cardiac fibrosis is characterized by the accumulation of extracellular matrix in the myocardium and is an integral component of most cardiac pathologic conditions, such as myocardial infarction, pressure overload, hypertrophic cardiomyopathy and dilated cardiomyopathy, and metabolic disturbances including diabetes and obesity. Following acute myocardial infarction, the death of cardiomyocytes triggers an inflammatory reaction, ultimately leading to the replacement of the dead myocardium with a collagen-based scar.

Endothelial-mesenchymal transition (EndMT) is a critical process that enhances the progression of fibrosis in the heart, where endothelial genes/proteins are decreasingly expressed and mesenchymal genes/proteins are increasingly expressed. It was reported that cardiac fibroblasts stimulated with EPC-EVs showed increased expression of EC-specific markers, such as CD31 and VEGF-2, and decreased expression of proteins involved in fibrosis, such as α-SMA, vimentin, collagen I, TGF-β, TNF-α, and HMGB1, thus promoting the proliferation and angiogenesis of cardiac fibroblasts by the EV-mediated inhibition of EndMT [56]. Further evidence also suggested that human EPC-EVs can promote the expression of endothelial markers in human cardiac fibroblasts through the inhibition of EndMT [56]. miRNAs are critical regulators involved in the activation of cardiac fibroblasts [57, 58] by EndMT [59]. Based on this, Lin et al. cultured rat cardiac fibroblasts with EVs derived from H/R-treated EPCs and demonstrated a significant up-regulation of miR-133 and increased expression of endothelial markers in fibroblasts, which suggested that EPC-EVs attenuated cardiac fibrosis via promoting fibroblast angiogenesis and MEndoT through the EV-mediated transfer of miR-133 [60]. Additionally, EVs from endothelial colony-forming cells under hypoxia significantly improved the mesenchymal to endothelial transition (MEndoT) in cardiac fibroblasts via reducing miR-10b-5p [42]. Those findings suggest that EPC-EVs could be employed as a therapeutic tool against fibroblast activation and endothelial-mesenchymal transition in cardiac fibrosis.

Angiogenesis

Angiogenesis is the process by which new capillary blood vessels form from pre-existing ones, which have the potential to repair the ischemic myocardium following myocardial infarction. Studies have shown that EPC–derived EVs exert beneficial effects, including the promotion of neovascularization and attenuation of ventricular wall thinning, and can be a new therapeutic method for CVDs. EPC-EVs can be applied to endothelial cells to enhance the cell proliferation and migration *in vitro* and promote vascular repair in rat models of balloon injury [61]. Further studies demonstrated that EPC-EVs could inhibit neointimal hyperplasia after carotid artery injury through the promotion of EC repair rather than the direct suppression of proliferation and migration of smooth muscles cells [62]. Additionally, promising results suggest that the administration of EPC-EVs enhanced re-endothelialization after endothelial damage via shuttling miR-21-5p [63]. A recent study reported that EPC-EVs with overexpression of miR-126 promoted angiogenesis and neurogenesis as well as neurological functional recovery in a diabetic mouse model of ischemic stroke [64]. Moreover, several studies suggested that EPC-EVs can enhance peri-infarct angiogenesis and hemodynamics after MI [65]. These studies suggest that EVs contain important bioactive molecules that can promote angiogenesis and induce protection against ischemia. Therefore, the promotion of neovascularization is a potential therapeutic approach for the treatment of CVDs with EPC-derived EVs.

Therapeutic Effects of EPC-derived EVs in the Treatment of Cardiovascular Diseases

The heart is composed of different cell types, including cardiomyocytes, fibroblasts, endothelial cells, smooth muscle cells, immune cells, and cardiac-derived stem cells. All these cells are organized in a complex structure and require balance to ensure the integrity of the heart. Intercellular communication is crucial in maintaining the balance between heart cells. Intercellular communication can be mediated through cell-cell contact, cell-matrix interaction, long-distance signals, and extracellular electric or biochemical signals [65-67]. Recently, more and more attention was focused on EVs mediating intercellular communication to local neighboring cells or distant organs [67-69]. Indeed, EVs and EV-contained microRNAs play a substantial role in various processes involved in the pathogenesis of cardiovascular diseases, such as myocardial infarction, ischemia/reperfusion injury, atherosclerosis, and cardiomyopathy [70-74].

Myocardial Infarction

Myocardial infarctions (MI) occur as a result of perfusion imbalance of oxygen and metabolic substrates [75, 76] between the supply and demand in cardiomyocytes caused by a partial or complete blockage of epicardial coronary arteries [77]. In general, cell death, including apoptosis, pyroptosis, and necrosis, occurs within 20 min of occlusion of coronary arteries; complete necrosis happens at 2–4 h after persistent or intermittent coronary arterial occlusion [78]. Without blood to supply cardiomyocytes, inflammatory changes in the cells also occur and this process occurs simultaneously as cardiomyocytes struggle to survive or die. Notably, the extracellular micro-environment, including extracellular matrix and extracellular vesicles, is greatly affected by MI, and vice versa [79, 80].

With the emergence of studies on EVs, EPC-derived EVs have been regarded to provide protective functions in CVDs. The early studies reported by Sahoo et al. demonstrated the therapeutic potential of EVs produced by human CD34+ EPCs in cardiovascular diseases [38, 81]. The authors observed that EVs isolated from CD34+ EPC showed similar angiogenic activity as CD34+ cells by enhancing the EC viability, proliferation, and tube formation on Matrigel *in vitro* and stimulating angiogenesis in Matrigel plug and corneal assays *in vivo*. Further studies found that EPC-EVs are enriched with proangiogenic miRNAs such as miR-126-3p, whereas knocking down miR-126-3p abolished the angiogenic activity and therapeutic effects of EPC-EVs both in vitro and in vivo [82]. Notably, cell internalization of EPC-EVs was observed to take place mostly in EC relative to smooth muscle cells and fibroblasts in hindlimb ischemic animal model, demonstrating a direct role of EPC-EVs on the endothelium at the cellular level. In a mouse MI model, EPC-EVs therapy significantly preserved the cardiac function, inhibited cell apoptosis, reduced MI scar size, and promoted neovascularization [83]. In contrast, the knockout of IL-10 in EPC-EVs showed diminished and opposite effects. Notably, the high expression of integrin-linked kinase (ILK) in IL-10 knockout EPC-EVs may be the potential mechanism for the dysfunction of these EVs. Another study utilizing an injectable hydrogel to deliver EPC-EVs into the ischemic myocardium also showed enhanced peri-infarct angiogenesis and myocardial hemodynamics, demonstrating the therapeutic efficiency and efficacy of EPC-EVs [65]. These works highlighted that EPC-EVs therapy presented very similar beneficial effects as the EPC treatment. The same group further reported that EPC-EVs in a shear thinning gel dramatically improved post-MI hemodynamics when delivered 4 days versus immediately post-infarct [84]. In addition, to regulate the functions of ECs, EPC-EVs were also found to attenuate the post-MI cardiac injury by promoting phenotypic changes of fibroblasts to endothelial cells through the exosomal transfer of miR-1246 and miR-1290 [85].

Reperfusion Injury

The restoration of blood supply to previously ischemic cardiac tissue may lead to metabolic disorders and myocardial dysfunction due to ROS production, calcium overload, and other changes, paradoxically causing further myocardial damage. Studies have shown that EPC-EVs injection after ischemia-reperfusion could significantly decrease the myocardial damage and preserve the heart function. The restoration of blood and oxygen supply cause ECs to produce a large amount of ROS associated with vascular dysfunction. It has been shown that treatment with EPC-EVs could dramatically decrease the apoptosis of ECs and attenuate excessive ROS production, leading to an improved EC function and neovascularization after hypoxia/reoxygenation (H/R) injury [54]. Further studies found that EPC-EVs can reduce EC apoptosis, ROS overproduction, and angiogenic dysfunction, and decrease mitochondrial fragmentation, which is boosted by miR-210 enrichment [54]. Moreover, Zhang et al. showed that EPC-EVs abundant miR-18a presented better protective effects on H/R injury in aging ECs via the down-regulation of the Nox2/ROS pathway. Thus, the transmission of miRNAs and subsequent gene silencing are important mechanisms through which EPC-EVs play a protective role.

Atherosclerosis

Atherosclerosis is the main underlying cause of cardiovascular disease characterized by endothelial dysfunction, intimal lipid deposition, smooth muscle cell proliferation, cell apoptosis and necrosis, and local and systemic inflammation [86]. Indeed, dysfunction of the endothelium is considered an early marker of atherosclerosis. Crosstalk mediated by EPC-derived EVs play an important role in the initiation, progression, and development of atherosclerosis. Alexandru et al. [87] studied the therapeutic effect of EPC-EVs on the atherosclerosis process: EPC-EVs were isolated from the peripheral blood of healthy hamsters and injected into hypertensive-hyperlipidemic hamsters through the retro-orbital sinus. The monthly EPC-EVs injection significantly alleviated the progress of atherosclerosis via modulating the circulating cytokine/chemokine levels, which in turn attenuated dyslipidemia, hypertension, and structural and functional remodeling. Another group [47] observed similar results: they reported that EPC-EVs could reduce atherosclerotic plaques and inflammatory factors, as well as ameliorate diabetic atherosclerosis endothelial dysfunction. Mechanistically, EPC-EVs abundant miR-199 was found to inhibit the ferroptosis of endothelial cells and subsequently alleviate the occurrence of atherosclerosis via targeting specificity protein 1 (SP1) [88].

Conclusion and Future Perspectives

The current isolation methods of EVs are primarily based on EV size, density, and surface markers. This heterogeneity of EVs hampers the biological characterization and therapeutic standardization, due to no available method or known specific marker to distinguish between exosomes and small microvesicles or between subpopulations. Relevant to the cardiovascular system, numerous modifications have been applied to maximize the beneficial effects of therapeutic EVs in ischemic heart diseases, hypoxic/ischemic injury, and inflammatory microenvironment. However, the preservation and delivery of biologically active cytokines, proteins, and miRNAs in EVs remain challenging for us. Since it is more attractive to use EPC-EVs as a therapeutic drug rather than conventional EPC transplantation, the biodistribution, long-term effects and safety of administered EPC-EVs would need to be studied and controlled.

Over the past decade, EVs have been extensively studied for its critical role in the therapeutic potential of cardiovascular diseases. EVs and their miRNA cargo will continue to represent an exciting therapeutic venue in the years to come for cardiovascular biology. Overall, cost- and time-effective technologies for large-scale production of EVs, further understanding of pathways involved in EV biogenesis, cargo loading, secretion. and uptake will be of fundamental importance to address how to alter the quality and quantity of EVs, as well as the therapeutic efficacy for the treatment of cardiovascular diseases.

Declaration of Competing Interest

The authors declare that there are no conflicts of interest.

References

[1] Shabbir A, Zisa D, Suzuki G, Lee T. Heart failure therapy mediated by the trophic activities of bone marrow mesenchymal stem cells: a noninvasive therapeutic regimen. *Am J Physiol Heart Circ Physiol.* 2009;296(6):H1888-97.

[2] Orlic D, Kajstura J, Chimenti S, Jakoniuk I, Anderson SM, Li B, et al. Bone marrow cells regenerate infarcted myocardium. *Nature.* 2001;410(6829):701-5.

[3] Stamm C, Westphal B, Kleine HD, Petzsch M, Kittner C, Klinge H, et al. Autologous bone-marrow stem-cell transplantation for myocardial regeneration. *Lancet.* 2003;361(9351):45-6.
[4] Asahara T, Murohara T, Sullivan A, Silver M, van der Zee R, Li T, et al. Isolation of putative progenitor endothelial cells for angiogenesis. *Science.* 1997;275(5302): 964-7.
[5] Asahara T, Chen D, Takahashi T, Fujikawa K, Kearney M, Magner M, et al. Tie2 receptor ligands, angiopoietin-1 and angiopoietin-2, modulate VEGF-induced post-natal neovascularization. *Circ Res.* 1998;83(3):233-40.
[6] Asahara T, Masuda H, Takahashi T, Kalka C, Pastore C, Silver M, et al. Bone marrow origin of endothelial progenitor cells responsible for postnatal vasculogenesis in physiological and pathological neovascularization. *Circ Res.* 1999;85 (3):221-8.
[7] Kalka C, Masuda H, Takahashi T, Gordon R, Tepper O, Gravereaux E, et al. Vascular endothelial growth factor (165) gene transfer augments circulating endothelial progenitor cells in human subjects. *Circ Res.* 2000;86(12):1198-202.
[8] Menasche P, Vanneaux V, Hagege A, Bel A, Cholley B, Cacciapuoti I, et al. Human embryonic stem cell-derived cardiac progenitors for severe heart failure treatment: first clinical case report. *Eur Heart J.* 2015;36(30):2011-7.
[9] Mauritz C, Martens A, Rojas SV, Schnick T, Rathert C, Schecker N, et al. Induced pluripotent stem cell (iPSC)-derived Flk-1 progenitor cells engraft, differentiate, and improve heart function in a mouse model of acute myocardial infarction. *Eur Heart J.* 2011;32(21):2634-41.
[10] Caspi O, Huber I, Kehat I, Habib M, Arbel G, Gepstein A, et al. Transplantation of human embryonic stem cell-derived cardiomyocytes improves myocardial performance in infarcted rat hearts. *J Am Coll Cardiol.* 2007;50(19):1884-93.
[11] Ohnishi S, Sumiyoshi H, Kitamura S, Nagaya N. Mesenchymal stem cells attenuate cardiac fibroblast proliferation and collagen synthesis through paracrine actions. *FEBS Lett.* 2007;581(21):3961-6.
[12] Zhao L, Liu X, Zhang Y, Liang X, Ding Y, Xu Y, et al. Enhanced cell survival and paracrine effects of mesenchymal stem cells overexpressing hepatocyte growth factor promote cardioprotection in myocardial infarction. *Exp Cell Res.* 2016;344 (1):30-9.
[13] Cocucci E, Meldolesi J. Ectosomes and exosomes: shedding the confusion between extracellular vesicles. *Trends Cell Biol.* 2015;25(6):364-72.
[14] Kalluri R, LeBleu VS. The biology, function, and biomedical applications of exosomes. *Science.* 2020;367(6478).
[15] Yanez-Mo M, Siljander PR, Andreu Z, Zavec AB, Borras FE, Buzas EI, et al. Biological properties of extracellular vesicles and their physiological functions. *J Extracell Vesicles.* 2015; 4:27066.
[16] Zaborowski MP, Balaj L, Breakefield XO, Lai CP. Extracellular Vesicles: Composition, Biological Relevance, and Methods of Study. *Bioscience.* 2015;65(8): 783-97.
[17] Raposo G, Stoorvogel W. Extracellular vesicles: exosomes, microvesicles, and friends. *J Cell Biol.* 2013;200(4):373-83.

[18] Wickman G, Julian L, Olson MF. How apoptotic cells aid in the removal of their own cold dead bodies. *Cell Death Differ.* 2012;19(5):735-42.

[19] Lafourcade C, Sobo K, Kieffer-Jaquinod S, Garin J, van der Goot FG. Regulation of the V-ATPase along the endocytic pathway occurs through reversible subunit association and membrane localization. *PLoS One.* 2008;3(7):0002758.

[20] Lange C, Prenninger S, Knuckles P, Taylor V, Levin M, Calegari F. The H(+) vacuolar ATPase maintains neural stem cells in the developing mouse cortex. *Stem Cells Dev.* 2011;20(5):843-50.

[21] Colombo M, Raposo G, Théry C. Biogenesis, secretion, and intercellular interactions of exosomes and other extracellular vesicles. *Annu Rev Cell Dev Biol.* 2014; 30:255-89.

[22] Hessvik NP, Llorente A. Current knowledge on exosome biogenesis and release. *Cell Mol Life Sci.* 2018;75(2):193-208.

[23] Wang C, Zhao T, Li Y, Huang G, White MA, Gao J. Investigation of endosome and lysosome biology by ultra pH-sensitive nanoprobes. *Adv Drug Deliv Rev.* 2017; 113: 87-96.

[24] Maas SLN, Breakefield XO, Weaver AM. Extracellular vesicles: unique intercellular delivery vehicles. *Trends Cell Biol.* 2017;27(3):172-88.

[25] Kowal J, Arras G, Colombo M, Jouve M, Morath JP, Primdal-Bengtson B, et al. Proteomic comparison defines novel markers to characterize heterogeneous populations of extracellular vesicle subtypes. *Proc Natl Acad Sci U S A.* 2016;113 (8): E968-77.

[26] Yoshioka Y, Konishi Y, Kosaka N, Katsuda T, Kato T, Ochiya T. Comparative marker analysis of extracellular vesicles in different human cancer types. *J Extracell Vesicles.* 2013;2.

[27] Jeppesen DK, Fenix AM, Franklin JL, Higginbotham JN, Zhang Q, Zimmerman LJ, et al. Reassessment of exosome composition. *Cell.* 2019;177(2):428-45.

[28] Murillo OD, Thistlethwaite W, Rozowsky J, Subramanian SL, Lucero R, Shah N, et al. exRNA atlas analysis reveals distinct extracellular rna cargo types and their carriers present across human biofluids. *Cell.* 2019;177(2):463-77.

[29] Chaput N, Thery C. Exosomes: immune properties and potential clinical implementations. *Semin Immunopathol.* 2011;33(5):419-40.

[30] Zhang Y, Liu Y, Liu H, Tang WH. Exosomes: biogenesis, biologic function and clinical potential. *Cell Biosci.* 2019; 9:19.

[31] Parizadeh SM, Jafarzadeh-Esfehani R, Ghandehari M, Parizadeh SMR, Hassanian SM, Rezayi M, et al. Circulating Exosomes as Potential Biomarkers in Cardiovascular Disease. *Curr Pharm Des.* 2018;24(37):4436-44.

[32] Ibrahim AG, Cheng K, Marban E. Exosomes as critical agents of cardiac regeneration triggered by cell therapy. *Stem Cell Reports.* 2014;2(5):606-19.

[33] Xitong D, Xiaorong Z. Targeted therapeutic delivery using engineered exosomes and its applications in cardiovascular diseases. *Gene.* 2016;575(2 Pt 2):377-84.

[34] Das S, Halushka MK. Extracellular vesicle microRNA transfer in cardiovascular disease. *Cardiovasc Pathol.* 2015;24(4):199-206.

[35] Zhang Y, Hu YW, Zheng L, Wang Q. Characteristics and roles of exosomes in cardiovascular disease. *DNA Cell Biol.* 2017;36(3):202-11.

[36] King TF, McDermott JH. Endothelial progenitor cells and cardiovascular disease. *J Stem Cells.* 2014;9(2):93-106.

[37] Asahara T, Kawamoto A, Masuda H. Concise review: Circulating endothelial progenitor cells for vascular medicine. *Stem Cells.* 2011;29(11):1650-5.

[38] Sahoo S, Klychko E, Thorne T, Misener S, Schultz KM, Millay M, et al. Exosomes from human CD34(+) stem cells mediate their proangiogenic paracrine activity. *Circ Res.* 2011;109(7):724-8.

[39] Alexandru N, Andrei E, Niculescu L, Dragan E, Ristoiu V, Georgescu A. Microparticles of healthy origins improve endothelial progenitor cell dysfunction via microRNA transfer in an atherosclerotic hamster model. *Acta Physiol (Oxf).* 2017;221(4):230-49.

[40] Campagnolo L, Leahy A, Chitnis S, Koschnick S, Fitch MJ, Fallon JT, et al. EGFL7 is a chemoattractant for endothelial cells and is up-regulated in angiogenesis and arterial injury. *Am J Pathol.* 2005;167(1):275-84.

[41] Zhou Y, Li P, Goodwin AJ, Cook JA, Halushka PV, Chang E, et al. Exosomes from endothelial progenitor cells improve the outcome of a murine model of sepsis. *Mol Ther.* 2018;26(5):1375-84.

[42] Liu W, Zhang H, Mai J, Chen Z, Huang T, Wang S, et al. Distinct Anti-Fibrotic Effects of exosomes derived from endothelial colony-forming cells cultured under normoxia and hypoxia. *Med Sci Monit.* 2018; 24:6187-99.

[43] Ma C, Wang J, Liu H, Chen Y, Ma X, Chen S, et al. Moderate exercise enhances endothelial progenitor cell exosomes release and function. *Med Sci Sports Exerc.* 2018;50(10):2024-32.

[44] Wang J, Liu H, Chen S, Zhang W, Chen Y, Yang Y. Moderate exercise has beneficial effects on mouse ischemic stroke by enhancing the functions of circulating endothelial progenitor cell-derived exosomes. *Exp Neurol.* 2020; 330: 113325.

[45] Kahroba H, Davatgaran-Taghipour Y. Exosomal Nrf2: From anti-oxidant and anti-inflammation response to wound healing and tissue regeneration in aged-related diseases. *Biochimie.* 2020;171-172:103-9.

[46] Mansoor H, Ong HS, Riau AK, Stanzel TP, Mehta JS, Yam GH. Current trends and future perspective of mesenchymal stem cells and exosomes in corneal diseases. *Int J Mol Sci.* 2019;20(12).

[47] Bai S, Yin Q, Dong T, Dai F, Qin Y, Ye L, et al. Endothelial progenitor cell-derived exosomes ameliorate endothelial dysfunction in a mouse model of diabetes. *Biomed Pharmacother.* 2020; 131:110756.

[48] Burger D, Vinas JL, Akbari S, Dehak H, Knoll W, Gutsol A, et al. Human endothelial colony-forming cells protect against acute kidney injury: role of exosomes. *Am J Pathol.* 2015;185(8):2309-23.

[49] Karmakar U, Chu JY, Sundaram K, Astier AL, Garside H, Hansen CG, et al. Immune complex-induced apoptosis and concurrent immune complex clearance are anti-inflammatory neutrophil functions. *Cell Death Dis.* 2021;12(4):296.

[50] Mirotsou M, Jayawardena TM, Schmeckpeper J, Gnecchi M, Dzau VJ. Paracrine mechanisms of stem cell reparative and regenerative actions in the heart. *J Mol Cell Cardiol.* 2011;50(2):280-9.

[51] Gnecchi M, Zhang Z, Ni A, Dzau VJ. Paracrine mechanisms in adult stem cell signaling and therapy. *Circ Res.* 2008;103(11):1204-19.

[52] Zhang C, Wang J, Ma X, Wang W, Zhao B, Chen Y, et al. ACE2-EPC-EXs protect ageing ECs against hypoxia/reoxygenation-induced injury through the miR-18a/Nox2/ROS pathway. *J Cell Mol Med.* 2018;22(3):1873-82.

[53] Wang J, Chen S, Bihl J. Exosome-mediated transfer of ACE2 (Angiotensin-Converting Enzyme 2) from endothelial progenitor cells promotes survival and function of endothelial cell. *Oxid Med Cell Longev.* 2020; 2020:4213541.

[54] Ma X, Wang J, Li J, Ma C, Chen S, Lei W, et al. Loading MiR-210 in endothelial progenitor cells derived exosomes boosts their beneficial effects on hypoxia/reoxygeneation-injured human endothelial cells via protecting mitochondrial function. *Cell Physiol Biochem.* 2018;46(2):664-75.

[55] Chen G, Li P, Liu Z, Zeng R, Ma X, Chen Y, et al. Enrichment of miR-126 enhances the effects of endothelial progenitor cell-derived microvesicles on modulating MC3T3-E1 cell function via Erk1/2-Bcl-2 signalling pathway. *Prion.* 2019;13(1): 106-15.

[56] Ke X, Yang D, Liang J, Wang X, Wu S, Wang X, et al. Human endothelial progenitor cell-derived exosomes increase proliferation and angiogenesis in cardiac fibroblasts by promoting the mesenchymal-endothelial transition and reducing high mobility group box 1 protein B1 expression. *DNA Cell Biol.* 2017;36(11):1018-28.

[57] Castoldi G, Di Gioia CR, Bombardi C, Catalucci D, Corradi B, Gualazzi MG, et al. MiR-133a regulates collagen 1A1: potential role of miR-133a in myocardial fibrosis in angiotensin II-dependent hypertension. *J Cell Physiol.* 2012;227(2):850-6.

[58] Bernardo BC, Gao XM, Winbanks CE, Boey EJ, Tham YK, Kiriazis H, et al. Therapeutic inhibition of the miR-34 family attenuates pathological cardiac remodeling and improves heart function. *Proc Natl Acad Sci U S A.* 2012;109(43): 17615-20.

[59] Ubil E, Duan J, Pillai IC, Rosa-Garrido M, Wu Y, Bargiacchi F, et al. Mesenchymal-endothelial transition contributes to cardiac neovascularization. *Nature.* 2014;514 (7524):585-90.

[60] Lin F, Zeng Z, Song Y, Li L, Wu Z, Zhang X, et al. YBX-1 mediated sorting of miR-133 into hypoxia/reoxygenation-induced EPC-derived exosomes to increase fibroblast angiogenesis and MEndoT. *Stem Cell Res Ther.* 2019;10(1):263.

[61] Li X, Chen C, Wei L, Li Q, Niu X, Xu Y, et al. Exosomes derived from endothelial progenitor cells attenuate vascular repair and accelerate reendothelialization by enhancing endothelial function. *Cytotherapy.* 2016;18(2):253-62.

[62] Kong J, Wang F, Zhang J, Cui Y, Pan L, Zhang W, et al. Exosomes of Endothelial Progenitor Cells Inhibit Neointima Formation After Carotid Artery Injury. *J Surg Res.* 2018; 232:398-407.

[63] Hu H, Wang B, Jiang C, Li R, Zhao J. Endothelial progenitor cell-derived exosomes facilitate vascular endothelial cell repair through shuttling miR-21-5p to modulate Thrombospondin-1 expression. *Clin Sci* (Lond). 2019;133(14):1629-44.

[64] Wang J, Chen S, Zhang W, Chen Y, Bihl JC. Exosomes from miRNA-126-modified endothelial progenitor cells alleviate brain injury and promote functional recovery after stroke. *CNS Neurosci Ther.* 2020;26(12):1255-65.

[65] Chen CW, Wang LL, Zaman S, Gordon J, Arisi MF, Venkataraman CM, et al. Sustained release of endothelial progenitor cell-derived extracellular vesicles from shear-thinning hydrogels improves angiogenesis and promotes function after myocardial infarction. *Cardiovasc Res.* 2018;114(7):1029-40.

[66] Pluchino S, Smith JA. Explicating exosomes: reclassifying the rising stars of intercellular communication. *Cell.* 2019;177(2):225-7.

[67] Mathieu M, Martin-Jaular L, Lavieu G, Théry C. Specificities of secretion and uptake of exosomes and other extracellular vesicles for cell-to-cell communication. *Nat Cell Biol.* 2019;21(1):9-17.

[68] Poe AJ, Knowlton AA. Exosomes and cardiovascular cell-cell communication. *Essays Biochem.* 2018;62(2):193-204.

[69] Sluijter JP, Verhage V, Deddens JC, van den Akker F, Doevendans PA. Microvesicles and exosomes for intracardiac communication. *Cardiovasc Res.* 2014;102 (2):302-11.

[70] Halkein J, Tabruyn SP, Ricke-Hoch M, Haghikia A, Nguyen NQ, Scherr M, et al. MicroRNA-146a is a therapeutic target and biomarker for peripartum cardiomyopathy. *J Clin Invest.* 2013;123(5):2143-54.

[71] Wang X, Huang W, Liu G, Cai W, Millard RW, Wang Y, et al. Cardiomyocytes mediate anti-angiogenesis in type 2 diabetic rats through the exosomal transfer of miR-320 into endothelial cells. *J Mol Cell Cardiol.* 2014; 74:139-50.

[72] Wu T, Chen Y, Du Y, Tao J, Zhou Z, Yang Z. Serum Exosomal MiR-92b-5p as a Potential Biomarker for Acute Heart Failure Caused by Dilated Cardiomyopathy. *Cell Physiol Biochem.* 2018;46(5):1939-50.

[73] Yang KC, Yamada KA, Patel AY, Topkara VK, George I, Cheema FH, et al. Deep RNA sequencing reveals dynamic regulation of myocardial noncoding RNAs in failing human heart and remodeling with mechanical circulatory support. *Circulation.* 2014;129(9):1009-21.

[74] Gallet R, Dawkins J, Valle J, Simsolo E, de Couto G, Middleton R, et al. Exosomes secreted by cardiosphere-derived cells reduce scarring, attenuate adverse remodelling, and improve function in acute and chronic porcine myocardial infarction. *Eur Heart J.* 2017;38(3):201-11.

[75] Barile L, Moccetti T, Marbán E, Vassalli G. Roles of exosomes in cardioprotection. *Eur Heart J.* 2017;38(18):1372-9.

[76] Kanamori H, Takemura G, Goto K, Maruyama R, Tsujimoto A, Ogino A, et al. The role of autophagy emerging in postinfarction cardiac remodelling. *Cardiovasc Res.* 2011;91(2):330-9.

[77] White HD, Chew DP. Acute myocardial infarction. *Lancet.* 2008;372(9638):570-84.

[78] Thygesen K, Alpert JS, White HD, Jaffe AS, Apple FS, Galvani M, et al. Universal definition of myocardial infarction. *Circulation.* 2007;116(22):2634-53.

[79] Alibhai FJ, Tobin SW, Yeganeh A, Weisel RD, Li RK. Emerging roles of extracellular vesicles in cardiac repair and rejuvenation. *Am J Physiol Heart Circ Physiol.* 2018;315(4):H733-H44.

[80] Frangogiannis NG. The extracellular matrix in myocardial injury, repair, and remodeling. *J Clin Invest.* 2017;127(5):1600-12.

[81] Sahoo S, Losordo DW. Exosomes and cardiac repair after myocardial infarction. *Circ Res.* 2014;114(2):333-44.

[82] Mathiyalagan P, Liang Y, Kim D, Misener S, Thorne T, Kamide CE, et al. Angiogenic mechanisms of human cd34(+) stem cell exosomes in the repair of ischemic hindlimb. *Circ Res.* 2017;120(9):1466-76.

[83] Yue Y, Wang C, Benedict C, Huang G, Truongcao M, Roy R, et al. Interleukin-10 deficiency alters endothelial progenitor cell-derived exosome reparative effect on myocardial repair via integrin-linked kinase enrichment. *Circ Res.* 2020;126(3):315-29.

[84] Chung JJ, Han J, Wang LL, Arisi MF, Zaman S, Gordon J, et al. Delayed delivery of endothelial progenitor cell-derived extracellular vesicles via shear thinning gel improves postinfarct hemodynamics. *J Thorac Cardiovasc Surg.* 2020;159(5):1825-35 e2.

[85] Huang Y, Chen L, Feng Z, Chen W, Yan S, Yang R, et al. EPC-derived exosomal miR-1246 and miR-1290 regulate phenotypic changes of fibroblasts to endothelial cells to exert protective effects on myocardial infarction by targeting ELF5 and SP1. *Front Cell Dev Biol.* 2021; 9:647763.

[86] Herrero-Fernandez B, Gomez-Bris R, Somovilla-Crespo B, Gonzalez-Granado JM. Immunobiology of Atherosclerosis: a complex net of interactions. *Int J Mol Sci.* 2019;20(21).

[87] Alexandru N, Andrei E, Safciuc F, Dragan E, Balahura AM, Badila E, et al. Intravenous administration of allogenic cell-derived microvesicles of healthy origins defend against atherosclerotic cardiovascular disease development by a direct action on endothelial progenitor cells. *Cells.* 2020;9(2).

[88] Li L, Wang H, Zhang J, Chen X, Zhang Z, Li Q. Effect of endothelial progenitor cell-derived extracellular vesicles on endothelial cell ferroptosis and atherosclerotic vascular endothelial injury. *Cell Death Discov.* 2021;7(1):235.

Editors' Contact Information

Amankeldi A. Salybekov, MD, PhD
Senior Clinical Researcher
PI at Clinical Research Center
Shonan Kamakura General Hospital
Kamakura, Japan
Email: a.salybekov@shonankamakura.or.jp

Dr. Shuzo Kobayashi, MD, PhD
Kidney Diseases and Transplant Center
Shonan Kamakura General Hospital
Kamakura, Japan
Email: shuzo@shonankamakura.or.jp

Dr. Takayuki Asahara, MD, PhD
Shonan Research Institute of Innovative Medicine
Fujisawa, Japan
Email: t_asahara@shonankamakura.or.jp

Index

D

E

L

M

N

O

P

Q

R

S

T

V